brain stars

glia illuminating craniosacral therapy

written and illustrated by Tad Wanveer, LMBT, CST-D

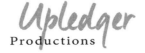

Copyright © 2015 Tad Wanveer. All rights reserved.

No part of this publication may be reproduced, stored in a retrieval system, or transmitted in any form or by any means, electronic, mechanical, photocopying, recording or otherwise, without the prior permission of the Publisher. Permissions may be sought directly from Upledger Productions Rights Department. Inquiries may be made by mail at 11211 Prosperity Farms Road, Suite D-325, Palm Beach Gardens, Florida, USA, 33410; phone at 561.622.4334; or e-mail at info@upledger.com.

ISBN: 978-0-9907966-1-9

Upledger Productions
11211 Prosperity Farms Road, Suite D-325
Palm Beach Gardens,
Florida, 33410
561.622.4334
www.upledger.com

Notice:
Neither the Publisher nor the Author assume any responsibility for any loss or injury and/or damage to persons or property arising out of, or related to, any use of the material contained in this book. It is the responsibility of the treating practitioner, relying on independent expertise and knowledge of the patient, to determine the best treatment and method of application for the patient.

Illustrator: Tad Wanveer
Cover illustrator: Tad Wanveer
Proofreader: Kathleen Fox
Indexer: WordCo Indexing Services

Upledger Productions
Your source for educational excellence.
www.Upledger.com

Printed in the U.S.A.

Preface

*B*rain stars are not in a far-away sky. They are within each person, just inside the bony cranium.

We each have billions of star-shaped cells in our brain. Brain stars are part of a family of cells called "glia." Glia and neurons create our inner universe of sensation, perception, memory, and action. Reaching inward…we can gently touch them.

How do craniosacral therapy (CST) techniques reach into the brain or spinal cord? Is there a biomechanical pathway through which CST corrective techniques are transmitted from a practitioner's hands into the depths of the central nervous system (CNS)? If so, what cells form this corrective pathway, what do they do, and how do they help CNS healing and function? The answer to all of these questions may reside in glia.

The purpose of this book is to show how glial cells:
- build a therapeutic interface from outside the CNS to inside the CNS,
- generate cerebrospinal fluid (CSF) and regulate CSF flow,
- contribute to CNS development,
- sustain and help govern the work of neurons,
- form glial communication systems,
- insulate CNS nerve fibers,
- help the CNS heal,
- transmit visual information,
- insulate peripheral nerves, and
- participate in sensory and autonomic nervous system processing.

Thank you,
Tad

Foreword
by Scott Forman, MD

Tad Wanveer has brought the practice of craniosacral therapy to a deeper level. Making us aware of the vast, heretofore unknown contribution of glial cells to neurophysiology, neuron cell metabolism, and synaptic transmission, he has deepened our understanding of the brain.

He delves into the complexities of the blood-brain barrier and the various routes cerebrospinal fluid travels from its conception to its re-absorption. Incorporating glial cells as the "guardians" of the barriers and their importance in cerebrospinal fluid production and metabolism, he brings our level of understanding to a new realm.

When we have these concepts formed in our left brain, it allows our hands to search for a deeper understanding of the client's mind and spirit. The greater our foundation of understanding is, from a viewpoint of cellular physiology, the more our creativity (right brain) can offer toward healing.

John E. Upledger, DO, OMM, scoured science journals on a daily basis. With his love of cellular physiology and its own beauty, he sought to bring together the essence of the cell with the spirit and soul, which he held in his hands to blend with the client.

Tad's book has carried through the principles set forth by Dr. Upledger. It is a joy to read. His illustrations bring out, in simple drawings, the complexity of the inter-relations of the glia, the cerebrospinal fluid, and all the other fluid compartments and membranes of this beautiful organ, the brain.

Thank you, Tad, for bringing this to us and honoring the concepts Dr. Upledger taught us to uphold. This book is a wonderful addition to the craniosacral therapist's library.

Table of contents

Preface .... *iii*

Foreword .... *v*

Dedication .... *viii*

Acknowledgments .... *ix*

1. Introduction and a few key words 1
2. Glial cell summary 9
3. The craniosacral system and its glial components 13
4. The pia-glial interface 33
5. Cerebrospinal fluid and its glial connection 57
6. Radial glia and central nervous system development ... 103
7. Astrocyte overview 117
8. Neurons, synapses, and astrocytes 129
9. The extracellular space and transmission types 161
10. The blood-brain barrier and the neurovascular unit 179
11. Oligodendrocytes and myelin 195
12. Microglia, microgliosis, and astrogliosis 203
13. Retinal glia 227
14. Peripheral nervous system glia 237

Bibliography 269

Index 287

This book is dedicated with heartfelt gratitude to

John E. Upledger, DO, OMM

Acknowledgments

I am deeply grateful and thankful to the following people:
- my wife, Joanie, and our family: Paul, William, Sabrina, Sarah, Brennan, and Kyle, for your constant love and support during this book-writing adventure;
- Sue Cotta, PT, MSPT, CST; Cathy Schneider, MA, CST, LMT; Lisa Schuster, LMT; and Mindy Totten, LMBT, CST-D, for your brilliant edits and suggestions that refined and expanded this book;
- Scott Forman, MD, for writing the foreword;
- Sue Cotta, PT, MSPT, CST, for writing the back cover testimonial;
- Katherine J. Cosmas; Rebecca Flowers, OTR, BCP, CST-D; Jackie Hand, LMBT, CMT, CST; Dawn Langnes, BS, LMT; Diego Maggio, DO, BSc (Hons), CST-D; Emmanuel Roche, PhD; Jie Roche, CST, PT; Shyamala Strack, OTR/L, CST-D; John Matthew Upledger; Lisa Upledger, DC, CST-D, FIAMA; Lisa Werness, CST, CFP; and Kathy Woll, BS, MBA, for your help and contributions to this book.

Chapter 1

Introduction and a few key words

The central nervous system (CNS) consists of the brain and spinal cord, two very delicate structures that are protected by the bony cranium and vertebral column. They are also encased within the craniosacral system (CSS), which surrounds, protects, nourishes, and cleanses the CNS. Glial cells form an interconnected structural and functional matrix throughout the entire CNS that is fused to the CSS. Glia also encase CNS neurons and blood vessels forming a neuro-glial-vascular network.

The function of glial cells was once thought to be primarily as providing structural support; they were seen as the glue which held neural networks together. However, research over the past 35 years has shown that glial cells are essential partners of neurons in nearly every aspect of CNS development, function, homeostasis, and healing.

More than glue

The CNS is dependent upon neuro-glial-vascular interactions to perform such critical functions as:
- CNS development,
- synapse formation,
- neural signaling and neural modulation,
- brain and spinal cord immune response,
- cerebral blood flow regulation,
- cerebrospinal fluid production and flow,
- CNS cleansing,
- CNS dysfunction or disease,
- CNS healing, and
- short- and long-term memory processing.

Glia are also major components of the peripheral nervous system (PNS), in which they are involved in tasks such as:
- motor signaling,
- insulating axons,
- sensory signaling,
- healing of injured neurons, and
- autonomic nervous system interactions.

Glia of both the CNS and PNS are discussed in following chapters. The craniosacral system (CSS) is also discussed in Chapter 3, "The craniosacral system and its glial components."

Glia keep neurons alive

Craniosacral Therapy (CST) is a light-touch manual therapy. One primary goal of CST is to help the body improve CNS function by lessening harmful structural strain of the craniosacral system (CSS).

Neurons and glia live and function within an environment maintained by glia. I believe one important route by which CST stimulates nervous system health and healing is by lessening adverse glial stress. For example, glia are key components in the production of cerebrospinal fluid (CSF), as well as in the regulation of CSF flow into and out of the CNS. If CSF production is altered, then CNS tissue may become starved of vital substances, such as water. If CSF flow becomes stifled, then debris, toxins, or other harmful substances build up in the CNS.

The CNS may be driven toward dysfunction because glia become overly stressed, toxic, or overwhelmed due to a lack of vital substances and a harmful cell environment. Eventually, neurons and glia suffer and may perish because glia can no longer efficiently support, protect, heal, or cleanse the CNS terrain.

How can we touch glia?

Glial cells and neurons form an interdependent structural and functional system throughout the CNS that is fused to the CSS. This fusion takes place where glial cells attach to the pia mater membrane. The pia mater membrane is the innermost membrane layer of the CSS. It interconnects with the other CSS membrane layers (meninges), and these layers connect to the bones of the cranium and spinal column. This bone-to-membrane-to-glial matrix is a dynamic biomechanical pathway CST practitioners can use to help their clients correct nervous system dysfunction (Figure 1.1). This pathway is discussed in Chapter 4, "The pia-glial interface."

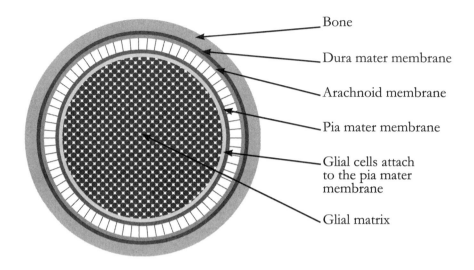

Figure 1.1 Diagram of the CNS showing the interconnection between bone and the glial matrix.

Key words

I have tried to make each chapter stand alone although there are times in which glial terminology is not redefined in each chapter.

There are a few words that will be helpful to define right now, they are:
- parenchyma,
- glial limiting membranes, and
- interstitium.

Parenchyma

"Parenchyma" means the specific tissue of an organ. In regards to the CNS, it is the tissue inside the pia mater membrane (Figure 1.2).

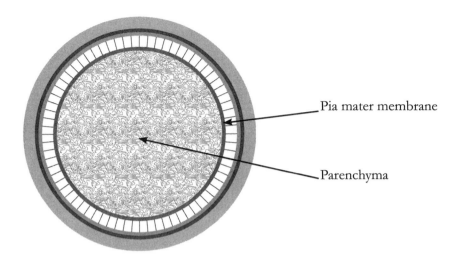

Figure 1.2. Diagram of the CNS showing the parenchyma inside the pia mater membrane.

Glial limiting membranes

There are three glial limiting membranes (Figure 1.3):
- outer glial limiting membrane,
- inner glial limiting membrane, and
- perivascular glial limiting membrane.

Outer glial limiting membrane

The outer glial limiting membrane is a membrane layer formed by glial processes that attach to the surface of the pia mater membrane facing the parenchyma (Figure 1.3).

Inner glial limiting membrane

The inner glial limiting membrane is a membrane layer formed by glial processes that attach to walls of the ventricular system facing the parenchyma (Figure 1.3).

Perivascular glial limiting membrane

The perivascular glial limiting membrane is formed by glial processes that surround all of the blood vessels within the parenchyma (Figure 1.3). The glial limiting membranes are discussed in a number of chapters, such as: Chapter 3, "The craniosacral system and its glial components;" Chapter 4, "The pia-glial interface;" and Chapter 5, "Cerebrospinal fluid and its glial connection."

Interstitium

"Interstitium" in the CNS is used to define areas within the boundaries formed by the three glial limiting membranes (Figure 1.3). Any substance entering or leaving the interstitium passes through a glial limiting membrane.

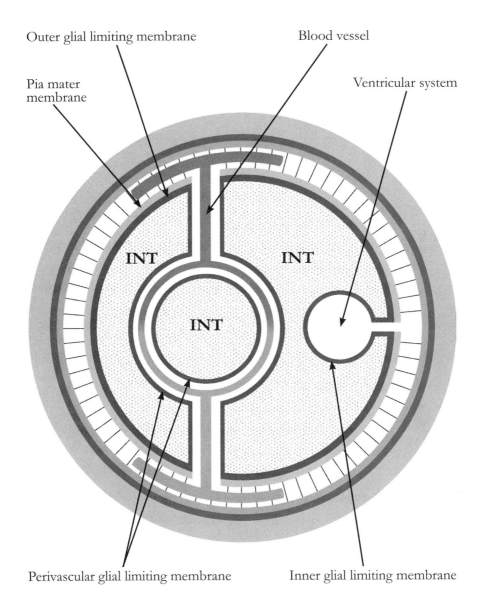

Figure 1.3. Diagram of the CNS showing the glial limiting membranes. "INT" identifies the interstitium.

Chapter 2

Glial cell summary

*I*n this chapter I will briefly describe cells that are discussed in subsequent chapters.

There are two classes of cells that make up the central nervous system (CNS): neurons and glia. Neurons comprise 10 percent of cells while glia comprise 90 percent. Glia are much smaller than neurons so the total CNS cell volume is 50 percent neurons and 50 percent glia.

Neurons

Neurons form circuits through which electrochemical signals are sent to coordinate complex body/mind processes by receiving, organizing, responding to, and storing neurological information.

Glial cells

Glial cells do not send signals in the same way neurons send signals, but they do communicate among themselves, as well as with neurons and blood vessels. Glial cells are involved in all aspects of CNS development, structure, function, health, and healing. For instance glial cells are:
- fundamental components in neuron information processing,
- interconnected cells that form a CNS-wide structural and communication matrix,
- CNS specialized immune cells,
- essential components of the blood-brain barrier,
- part of the neurovascular unit (the neurovascular unit regulates CNS blood flow), and
- primary elements of the craniosacral system.

CNS glia

There are three main types of glial cells in the CNS:
- astrocytes, which have a multitude of essential functions such as regulating the flow of cerebrospinal fluid;
- oligodendrocytes, which are myelinating cells; and
- microglia, which are specialized CNS immune cells.
    Other forms of glia exist, such as:
- ependymal cells that form the ventricles and part of the choroid plexuses;
- NG2 cells that are glial stem cells;
- radial glia, which are temporary glial cells that exist during prenatal development; and
- tanycytes, which convey information about cerebrospinal fluid to the hypothalamus and pituitary gland.

Peripheral nervous system glia

Glia are also part of the peripheral nervous system (PNS). Glia found in the PNS include:
- Schwann cells, which are myelinating cells;
- satellite cells of the sensory ganglia, which have similar functions as astrocytes;
- satellite cells of the autonomic ganglia, which have similar functions as astrocytes;
- enteric cells of the intestinal nervous system, which have similar functions as astrocytes; and
- olfactory ensheathing glia, which are cells encasing bundles of olfactory axons.

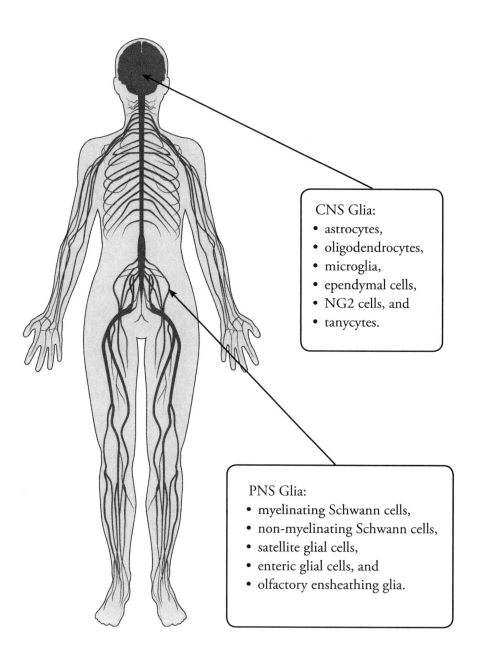

Figure 2.1. Glia of the CNS and PNS.

Chapter 3

The craniosacral system and its glial components

*I*n this chapter I will first describe the craniosacral system (CSS) and then discuss the glial cells that are essential components of the CSS.

The brain and spinal cord are very delicate and lack an internal connective tissue supportive matrix. They are protected by the bony cranium and spinal column and encased within the craniosacral system. The CSS surrounds, protects, nourishes, and cleanses the brain and spinal cord. It is comprised of:
- meninges,
- bones attaching to the meninges,
- cerebrospinal fluid (CSF), and
- CSS glia.

The meninges

The meninges consist of three connective tissue layers, also known as fascial layers, which encase both the brain and spinal cord (Figure 3.1 to Figure 3.3). The meningeal layers are the following:
- pia mater membrane,
- arachnoid membrane, and
- dura mater membrane.

Meningeal cell structure

Each meningeal layer consists of:
- cells that produce connective tissue (fibroblasts);
- connective tissue fibrous protein, such as collagen; and
- extracellular matrix.

The meninges encasing the brain

The pia mater membrane adheres to the surface of the brain tissue.

The arachnoid membrane surrounds the pia mater membrane. A CSF-filled space is found between the pia mater membrane and the arachnoid membrane. This space is called the "subarachnoid space."

"Trabeculae," which means "small beams," are fibroblasts spanning the subarachnoid space. They are extensions of the arachnoid membrane that attach to the pia mater membrane to help stabilize the subarachnoid space and maintain the position of blood vessels within the space.

The dura mater membrane surrounds and adheres to the arachnoid membrane. The dura mater membrane is comprised of two fascial layers fused to one another (Figure 3.4), they are the:
- meningeal layer, which adheres to the arachnoid membrane; and
- periosteal layer, which adheres to the bones of the cranial cavity forming the periosteum of the cranial bones.

CHAPTER 3 THE CRANIOSACRAL SYSTEM AND ITS GLIAL COMPONENTS

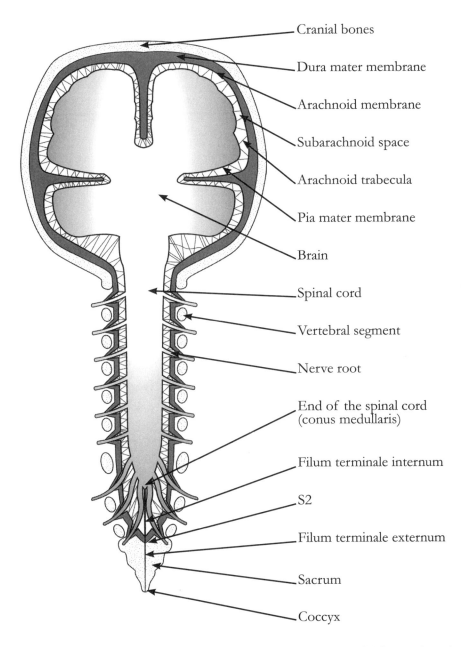

Figure 3.1. Anterior diagram of the meninges encasing the CNS. The meningeal layers encasing the spinal cord are referred to as the "dural sac." The dural sac ends at S2 where the three meningeal layers fuse together. These fused layers extend caudally where they blend with the fascia of the coccyx.

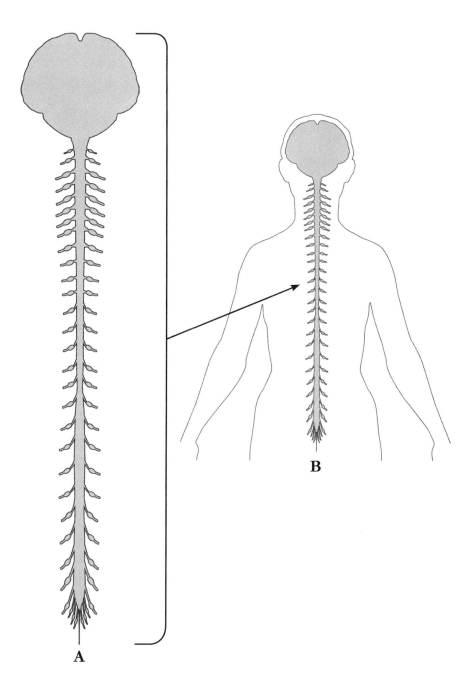

Figure 3.2. A: Anterior view of the dural sac and nerve roots. **B:** Dural sac within a figure.

CHAPTER 3   THE CRANIOSACRAL SYSTEM AND ITS GLIAL COMPONENTS

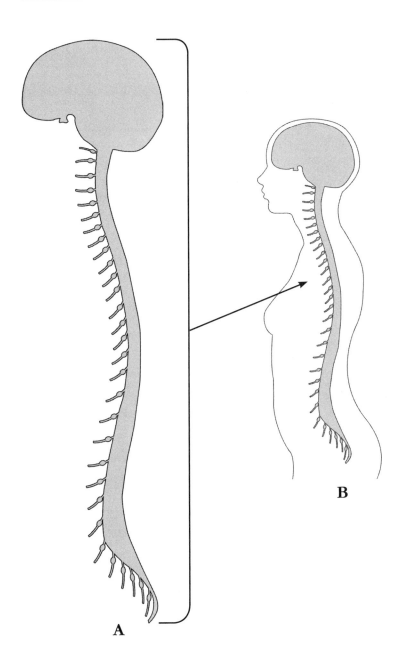

Figure 3.3. A: Lateral view of the dural sac and nerve roots. **B:** Dural sac within a figure.

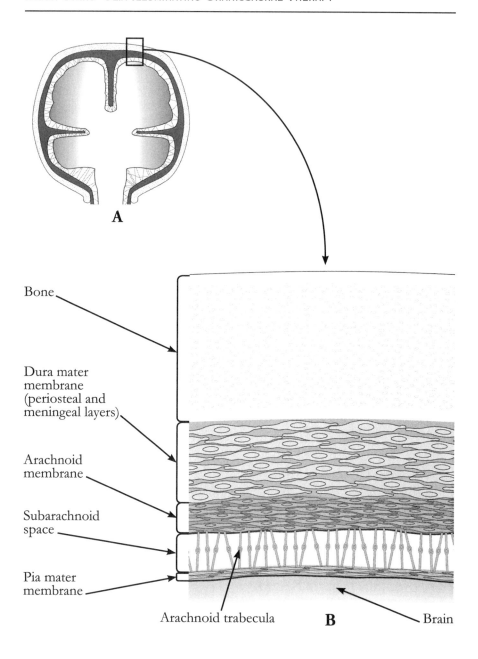

Figure 3.4. A: Anterior view of the meningeal layers surrounding the brain. **B:** Detail of the meningeal layers, subarachnoid space, and arachnoid trabeculae.

Infolding of the dura mater membrane and the arachnoid membrane

There are a few places where the meningeal layer separates from the periosteal layer to form fascial sheets that extend into the brain tissue. One of the sheets is arranged in a front-to-back (anterior-to-posterior) direction and is called the "falx cerebri and falx cerebelli." Another sheet arranged in a side-to-side (lateral-to-lateral) direction is called the "tentorium cerebelli." The arachnoid membrane follows the in-folded meningeal layers, and the pia mater membrane continues to adhere to the brain tissue surface (Figure 3.5 and Figure 3.6).

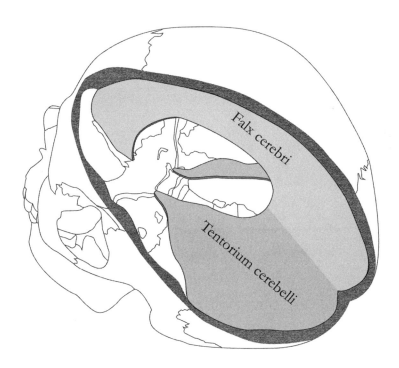

Figure 3.5. Left lateral 3/4 view of the in-folded meningeal layers.

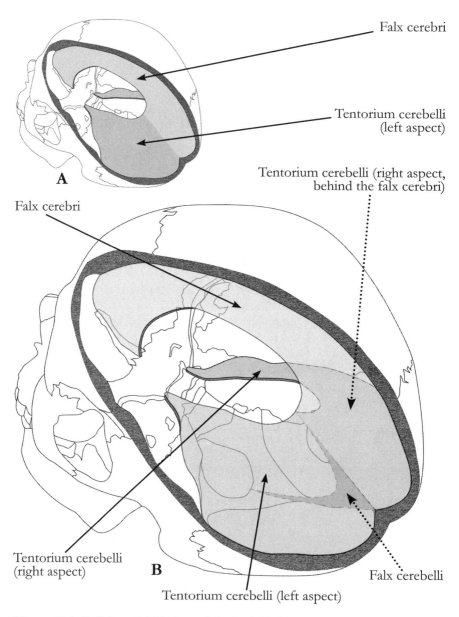

Figure 3.6. Left lateral 3/4 view of the in-folded meningeal layers. **A:** Opaque meningeal layers. **B:** Transparent meningeal layers. The meningeal layers are slightly transparent to show the falx cerebelli (dashed lines) underneath the tentorium cerebelli and a portion of the right aspect of the tentorium cerebelli (dashed lines) that is behind the falx cerebri.

The dural venous sinus system

The dural venous sinus system is an interconnected set of tubes (venous channels) within the cranium that drain venous blood and CSF out of the brain and spinal cord. It is formed within the cranial dura mater membrane (Figure 3.7).

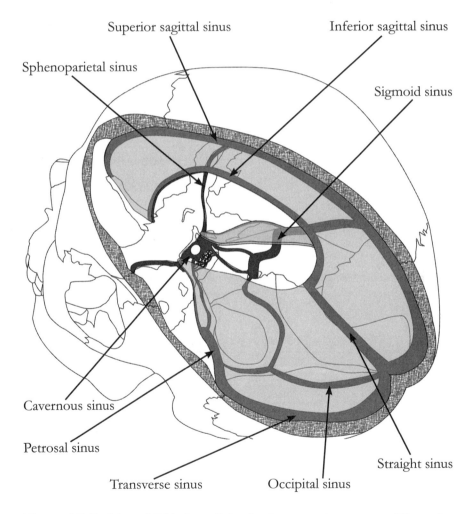

Figure 3.7. Left lateral 3/4 view of the dural venous sinus system. The major sinuses are identified.

Meninges encasing the spinal cord

The meninges encase the entire spinal cord and portions of the spinal nerve roots within the spinal canal and sacral canal (Figure 3.8).

The pia mater membrane adheres to the surface of the spinal cord and portions of the nerve roots. The arachnoid membrane adheres to the dura mater meningeal layer, and the CSF-filled subarachnoid space is found in between the pia mater membrane and arachnoid membrane.

The cranial dura mater membrane layers separate just below the foramen magnum. The dura mater periosteal layer merges with the periosteum of the spinal canal. The dura mater meningeal layer surrounds and adheres to the arachnoid membrane.

Between the wall of the spinal canal and the dura mater meningeal layer is the "epidural space." The epidural space is filled with adipose tissue forming a fatty tube around the meningeal layers encasing the spinal cord and portions of the nerve roots. Epidural adipose tissue helps to cushion and support the spinal cord while also allowing for a slight degree of mobility of the spinal cord within the spinal canal.

Bones attaching to the meninges

The periosteal layer of the dura mater membrane encasing the brain is attached to the bones of the cranial cavity (Figure 3.9).

The dura mater meningeal layer surrounding the spinal cord typically has the following bony attachments (Figure 3.9):
- foramen magnum (entire circumference);
- C2, C3, and S2 (anterior aspect is attached to the spinal canal); and
- coccyx.

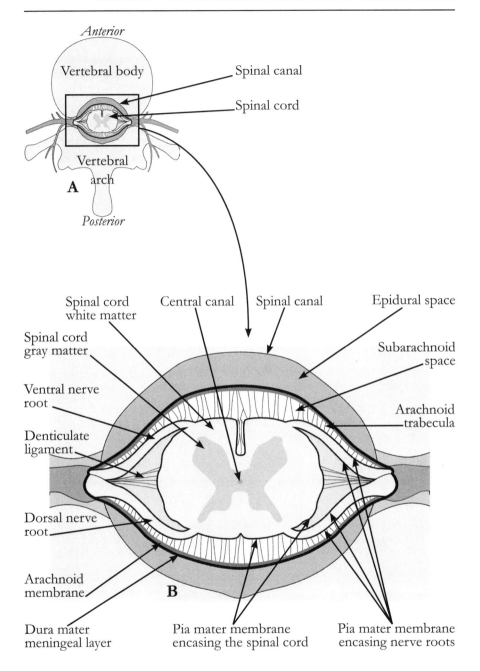

Figure 3.8. Spinal cord meningeal layers. **A:** Transverse section of the spinal column, spinal cord, and meninges. **B:** Transverse section detail of the meningeal layers surrounding the spinal cord and nerve roots.

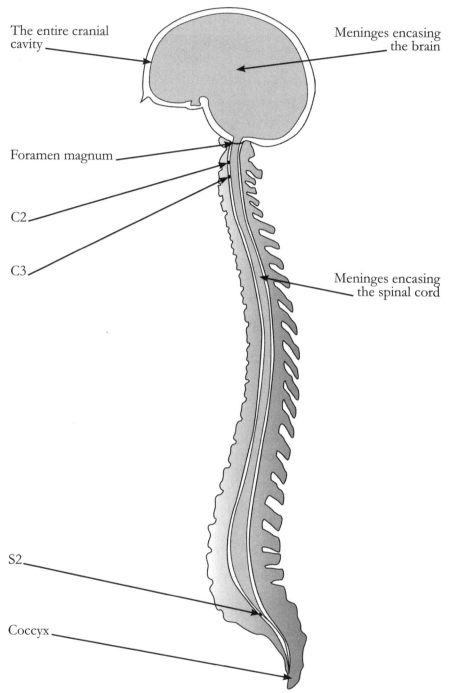

Figure 3.9. Lateral view showing the bony attachments of the dura mater membrane.

CSF

The following is a brief overview of CSF physiology. CSF is covered in detail in Chapter 5, "Cerebrospinal fluid and its glial connection."

CSF is formed from blood and is essential to the health of the CNS in a number of ways:
- protects the CNS from trauma by floating both the brain and spinal cord within a layer of CSF,
- lessens the effect of gravity on the brain (the adult brain weighs about 1500 grams, yet suspended in CSF it weighs about 50 grams);
- supplies vital nutrients,
- removes waste products, and
- helps maintain a stable and optimal CNS biochemical environment.

Freely flowing and precisely regulated CSF is indispensable to CNS health. Alterations in CSF production, composition, circulation, or pressure can adversely affect CNS function leading to disturbances of sensory, cognitive, or motor function.

A classical view of CSF production

CSF is produced within four interconnected cavities within the brain called "ventricles." Two of the ventricles are called "lateral ventricles" and the other two are referred to as the "third ventricle" and "fourth ventricle (Figure 3.10).

The lateral ventricles connect to the third ventricle by way of short channels called the "interventricular foramina" (also known as the "foramina of Monro"). The third ventricle is connected to the fourth ventricle by a slender channel called the "cerebral aqueduct." The fourth ventricle has a thin tube-like extension within the spinal cord where it is called the "central canal." The central canal extends within the middle of the spinal cord to the end of the spinal cord (conus medullaris).

A classical view of CSF flow from the ventricles into CNS tissue

CSF flows through the ventricles to the fourth ventricle. The fourth ventricle has three openings through which CSF flows into the subarachnoid space surrounding both the brain and the spinal cord. CSF then flows from the subarachnoid space into the CNS parenchyma by flowing through the pia mater membrane to provide CNS tissue with essential elements.

A classical view of CSF drainage

CSF picks up waste products and flows out of the CNS tissue into the subarachnoid space by diffusing through the pia mater membrane. CSF then flows through small valve-like extensions of the arachnoid membrane (arachnoid villi) to enter the dural venous sinus system. The dural venous sinus system transports CSF primarily to the jugular veins where CSF then flows into the body's general circulation.

CSF quantity and rate of renewal

The total amount of CSF within the ventricles and subarachnoid space of an adult typically equals 120-150 milliliters (about 4-5 ounces). Twenty-five percent (25%) is within the ventricles, and seventy-five percent (75%) is within the subarachnoid space. The total amount of CSF is normally renewed four to five times a day.

CSS glia

Glial cells are essential components of the CSS. The following is a very brief description of CSS glia. Detailed descriptions are found in Chapter 5, "Cerebrospinal fluid and its glial connection," and Chapter 7, "Astrocyte overview."

Ventricular system ependymal cells

The ventricles and their interconnecting channels are lined with glial cells called "ependymal cells" (Figure 3.10). Ependymal cells:
- secrete a small portion of CSF into the ventricles,
- help circulate CSF within the ventricles,
- help cleanse the inner surface of the ventricles of waste,
- form a barrier between intra-ventricular CSF and substances within the interstitium, and
- transport a small portion of CSF into the interstitium.

Choroid plexus ependymal cells

Each ventricle has a structure within it called a "choroid plexus," which is the site of most CSF production (Figure 3.10). A choroid plexus is comprised of a dense area of ependymal cells and capillaries, which together are referred to as the "blood-CSF barrier." Each choroid plexus filters and secretes elements from blood into the ventricles to form CSF.

CNS fluid barriers

CNS tissue is very delicate structurally and highly sensitive metabolically. The meninges, bony structures and CSF protect the CNS structurally. Metabolic protection is provided by four fluid-barrier systems:
- blood-CSF barrier,
- blood-brain barrier,
- glial limiting membranes, and
- subarachnoid space barriers.

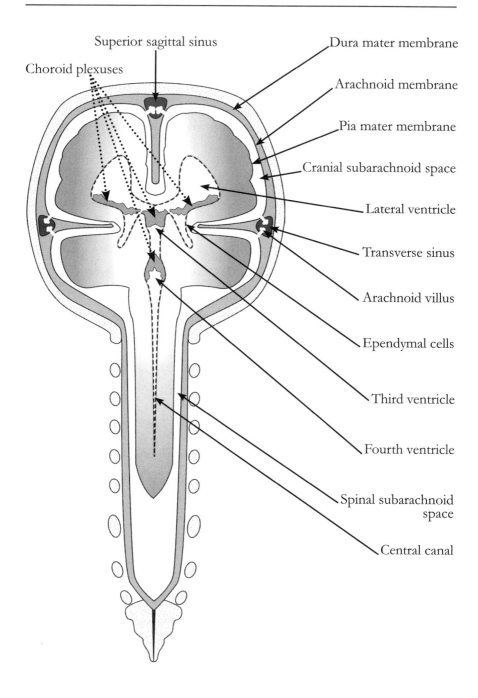

Figure 3.10. Anterior diagram of the ventricular system and the choroid plexuses.

Blood-CSF barrier

The blood-CSF barrier is briefly described above in the paragraph titled "Choroid plexus ependymal cells," and in detail in Chapter 5, "Cerebrospinal fluid and its glial connection."

Blood-brain barrier

The blood-brain barrier (BBB) is found throughout the entire parenchymal vascular system. The BBB is formed of blood vessels and the type of glial cells called "astrocytes." Astrocyte processes encase all parenchymal blood vessels. Substances entering the interstitium are regulated by the BBB. The BBB is covered in detail in Chapter 10, "The blood-brain barrier and the neurovascular unit."

Glial limiting membranes

Substances entering and leaving the CNS are regulated by astrocyte processes that form barriers, which are the following:
- outer limiting membrane that is attached to the side of the pia mater membrane facing towards the interstitium (Figure 3.11),
- inner glial limiting membrane that is attached to the surface of the ventricular system facing towards the interstitium (Figure 3.11), and
- perivascular glial limiting membrane that surrounds the entire parenchymal vascular system (Figure 3.11).

These glial membranes are described in detail in Chapter 5, "Cerebrospinal fluid and its glial connection;" and Chapter 7, "Astrocyte overview."

Subarachnoid space barriers

Astrocyte end-feet attached to the pia mater membrane are called the "outer glial limiting membrane." The outer limiting membrane plus the pia mater membrane form a barrier between the CNS parenchyma and the subarachnoid space. This keeps harmful substances that may be within the subarachnoid space from entering into the CNS parenchyma.

The arachnoid membrane forms a barrier between the subarachnoid space and the dura mater membrane (Figure 3.12). This assures that cerebrospinal fluid and subarachnoid space substances do not leak into the dura mater membrane. It also assures that substances in the dura mater membrane do not leak into the subarachnoid space, contaminating the contents of the subarachnoid space.

Glia interconnect the CSS with the entire CNS

Astrocytes form an interconnected cell matrix throughout the entire CNS. This matrix:
- surrounds almost all of the cells and structures within the interstitium,
- surrounds all parenchymal blood vessels, and
- attaches to the pia mater membrane, the walls of the ventricular system, and the walls of the central canal.

The astrocyte matrix forms a continuum extending from the bones encasing the CNS into the depths of the CNS. This interconnection is described in many sections of the book, including the following chapter, "The pia-glial interface."

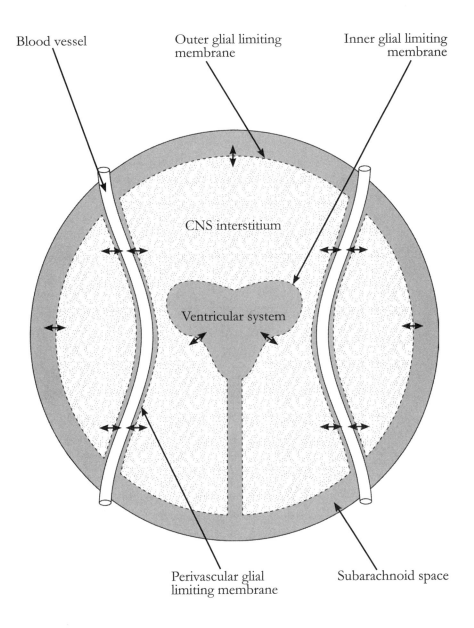

Figure 3.11. Diagram of the glial limiting membranes. The double-arrow line (↔) represents regulation by the glial limiting membranes of substances entering and leaving the CNS interstitium.

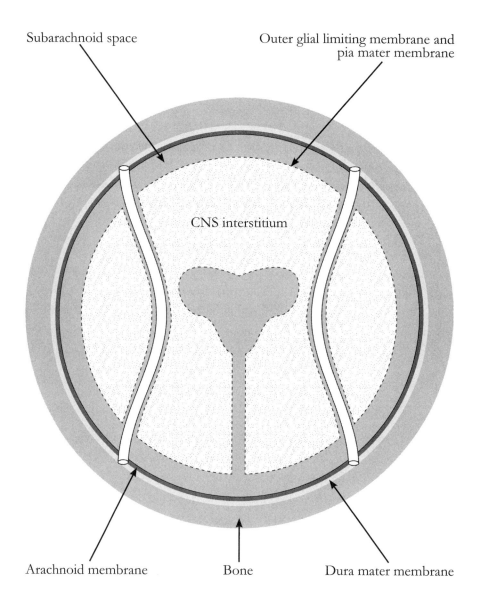

Figure 3.12. Diagram of the subarachnoid space barriers.

Chapter 4

The pia-glial interface

*H*ow does the application of craniosacral therapy (CST) facilitate central nervous system (CNS) correction? Lessening adverse stress of the craniosacral system membrane layers is said to help the CNS correct both structurally and functionally. How does this happen? It appears that the answer lies in the interconnection of the pia mater membrane with the outer glial limiting membrane. I call this interconnection the "pia-glial interface" (PGI). In this chapter we will discuss the PGI.

Fascia does not exist within the CNS parenchyma. However, fascial biomechanical forces can be transmitted into the CNS, and CNS biomechanical patterns can be transferred into fascia (Figure 4.1 to Figure 4.4). What links fascia and the parenchyma together?

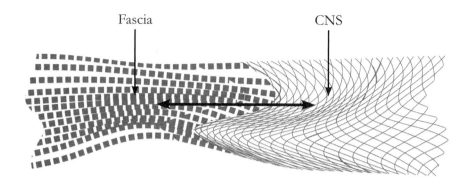

Figure 4.1. Transmission of biomechanical patterns between fascia and the CNS represented by ←——→.

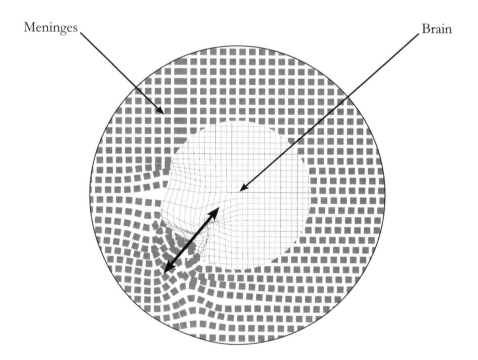

Figure 4.2. Transmission of biomechanical strain pattern between the meninges and the brain represented by ←——→.

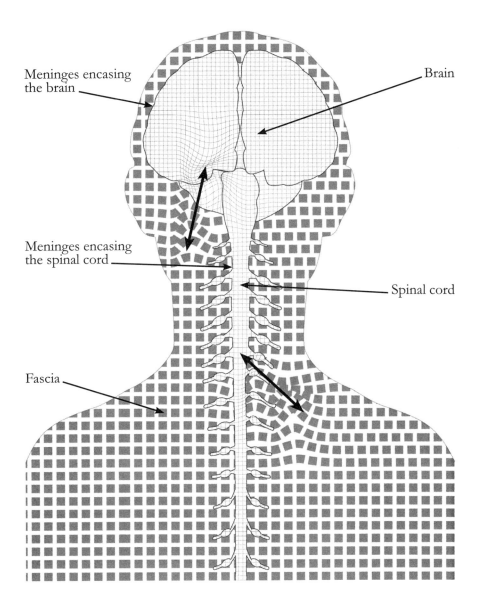

Figure 4.3. Transmission of biomechanical strain patterns between fascia and the CNS represented by ⟷.

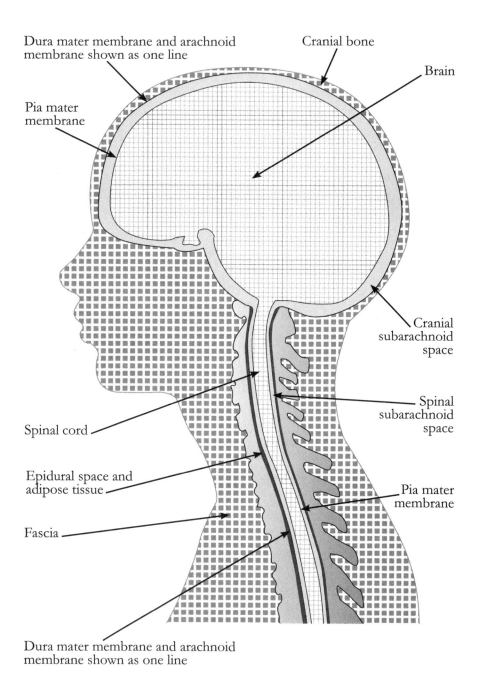

Figure 4.4. Lateral view of the brain and a portion of the spinal cord. Note: bone is classified as fascia in an expanded definition of fascia.

The PGI

The pia mater membrane is a meningeal layer adhering to the surface of the CNS. The outer surface of the CNS is covered by a very thin layer of extracellular matrix called the "basal lamina." CNS glial cells called "astrocytes" extend projections of their cell body outward to attach to the pia mater membrane. These astrocyte projections have slightly expanded tips, called "end-feet" (Figure 4.5). The combination of astrocyte end-feet and the CNS surface basal lamina is called the "outer glial limiting membrane." Astrocytes have many critical functions, and one appears to be responding to and transmitting biomechanical patterns.

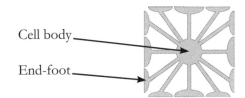

Figure 4.5. Schematic illustration of an astrocyte.

The the pia mater membrane-to-glial interconnection is a transition zone from outside to inside the CNS, and can be referred to as the "pia-glial interface" (PGI) (Figure 4.6).

The PGI is a structural boundary between fascia and the CNS where biomechanical patterns can be transferred from the:
- meninges into the outer glial limiting membrane,
- outer glial limiting membrane into the CNS parenchyma,
- CNS into the outer glial limiting membrane, and
- outer glial limiting membrane into the meninges (the meninges can transfer these patterns into the surrounding fascia).

In other words, the PGI is a two-way street through which stressful or corrective forces can move in two directions: outside to inside the CNS, and/or inside to outside the CNS (Figure 4.7 to Figure 4.15).

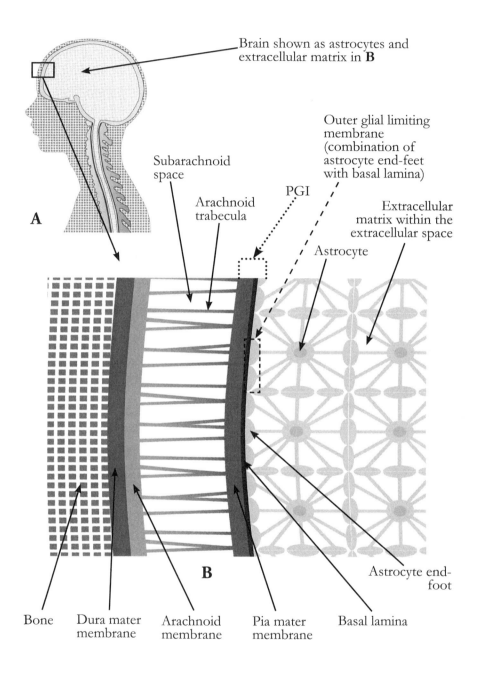

Figure 4.6. The PGL. **A:** Lateral view of the CNS. **B:** Detail of interconnection of bone to outer glial limiting membrane

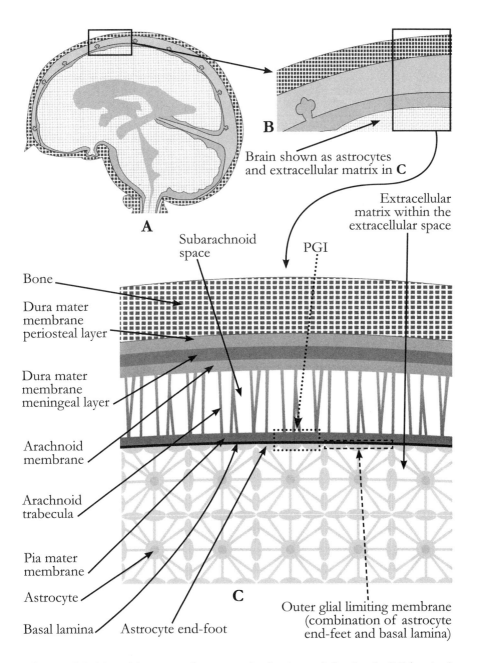

Figure 4.7. Transition zone between the brain and fascia. **A:** Midsagittal section of the brain. **B:** Detail of the meninges and brain. **C:** Detail of interconnection of bone to brain.

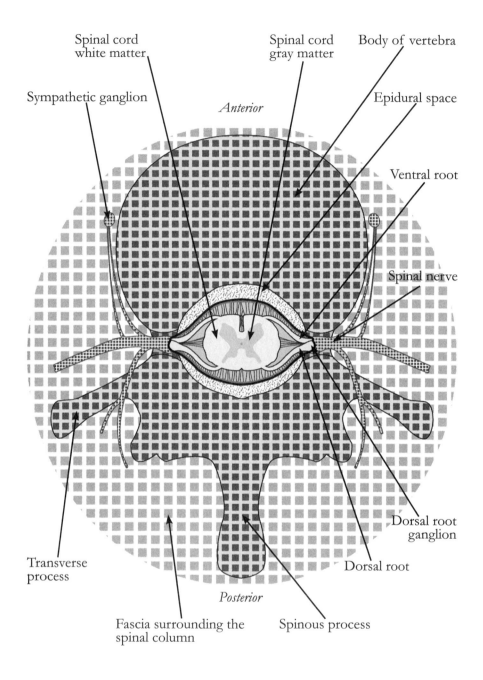

Figure 4.8. Transverse section of the vertebral column, spinal cord, and nerve roots showing continuum extending from fascia to spinal cord.

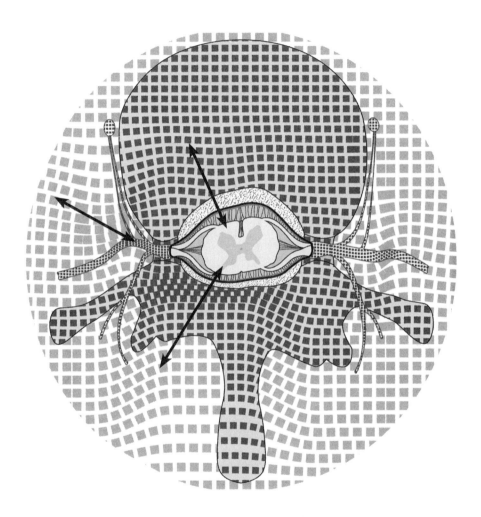

Figure 4.9. Fascial-glial matrix adverse strain. Transverse section showing the transfer of stressful biomechanical patterns between fascia, vertebral column, spinal cord, and nerve roots represented by ←→.

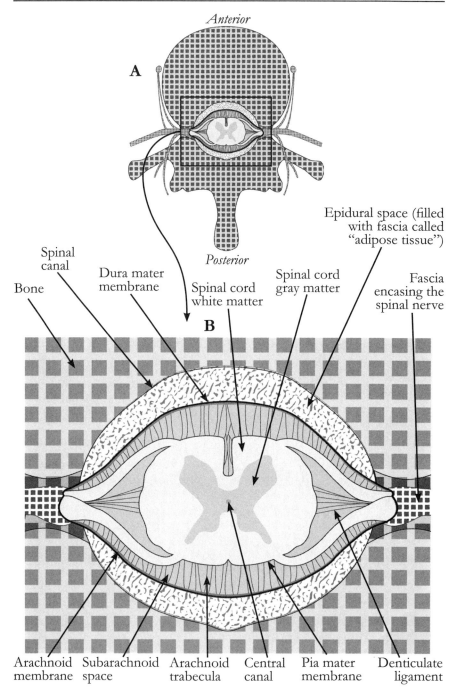

Figure 4.10. The spinal cord within the spinal canal. **A:** Transverse section of the spinal column and spinal cord. **B:** Detail of the spinal cord.

CHAPTER 4   THE PIA-GLIAL INTERFACE

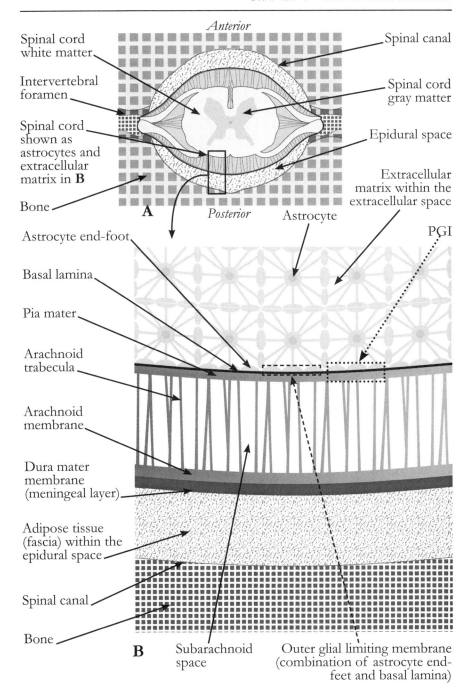

Figure 4.11. Transition zone between the spinal cord and fascia. **A:** Detail of the spinal cord. **B:** Detail of interconnection from bone to spinal cord.

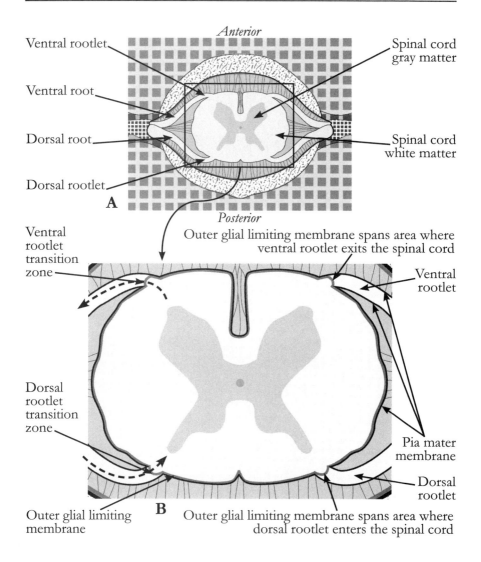

Figure 4.12. Spinal cord rootlet transition zone. **A:** Detail of the spinal cord. **B:** Detail of the spinal cord pia mater membrane and outer glial limiting membrane. The pia mater membrane encases rootlets as they exit or enter the spinal cord. The ventral rootlet transition zone is located where the outer glial limiting membrane spans across the area where ventral rootlet fibers exit the spinal cord. The dorsal rootlet transition zone is located where the outer glial limiting membrane spans across the area where dorsal rootlet fibers enter the spinal cord. Dashed arrows show direction of sensory input through the dorsal rootlet and motor output through the ventral rootlet.

CHAPTER 4   THE PIA-GLIAL INTERFACE

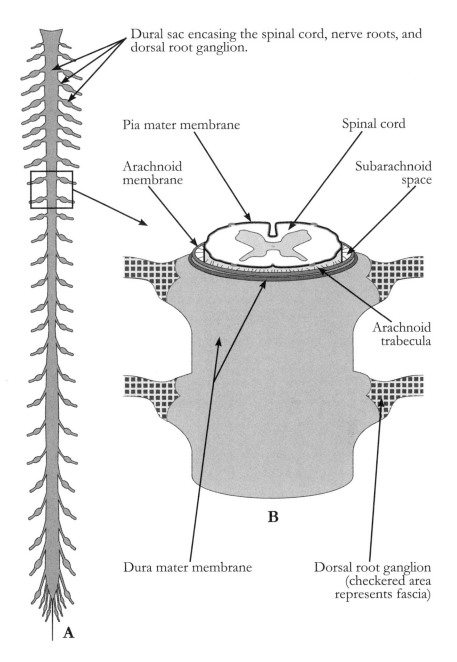

Figure 4.13. A: Posterior view of the dural sac encasing the spinal cord and nerve roots and dorsal root ganglia. **B:** Posterior detail of a portion of the dural sac and spinal cord.

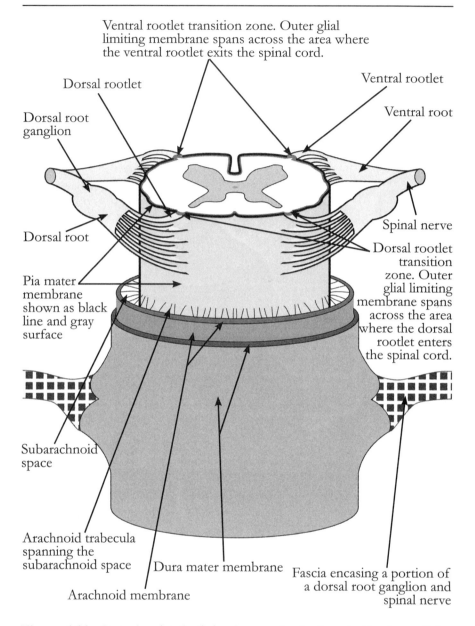

Figure 4.14. Posterior detail of dural sac and spinal cord. Portions of the meninges have been removed to show meningeal layers, nerve roots, nerve rootlets, and spinal cord. Each nerve root is a bundle of nerve fibers. Dorsal nerve roots give rise to smaller bundles of nerve fibers (dorsal nerve rootlets) that enter the spinal cord. Ventral nerve rootlets emerge from the spinal cord and join together to form ventral nerve roots.

Chapter 4   The pia-glial interface

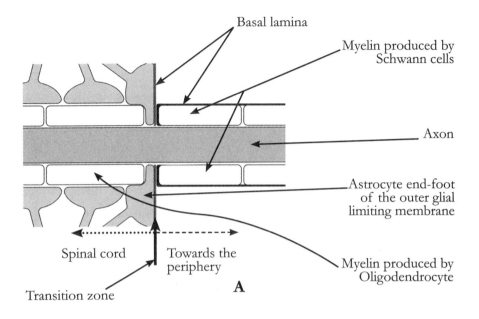

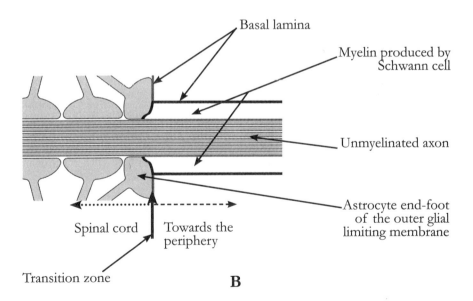

Figure 4.15. Rootlet transition zone. **A:** Detail of a myelinated nerve fiber rootlet transition zone. **B:** Detail of a non-myelinated nerve fiber rootlet transition zone.

Biomechanical transmission

Balanced and imbalanced biomechanical shape (BS) and corrective or stressful biomechanical forces (BF) can be transmitted through the fascial system all the way into the depths of the CNS. Disturbances of fascia can alter CNS structure by causing PGI distortions. These distortions can be transferred into the CNS parenchyma by deforming the outer glial limiting membrane, which then transmits these forces into the CNS.

Fascia transmits BS and BF through its extracellular matrix (ECM) structural fibrous proteins (such as, collagen and elastin), and through its ECM ground substance.

Since fascia does not exist in the CNS, it appears BS and BF are transmitted by astrocytes and CNS extracellular matrix ground substance. Astrocytes, the most abundant cells in the CNS, create an interconnected astrocyte network called the "glial syncytium." The glial syncytium extends throughout the entire CNS and it appears to have the capacity to transmit BS and BF throughout the CNS.

ECM in the CNS is a distinct substance and is produced by glia and neurons. CNS ECM composition is primarily ground substance, and it is fundamentally absent of structural fibrous proteins. CNS ECM ground substance has the capacity to transmit BS and BF.

PGI as a corrective interface

The interconnection of fascia with the CNS occurs through a reciprocal network of the PGI, glial syncytium, and ECM. Adverse strain in any part can impact the entire fascial-glial network to some extent. Conversely, correction of one part can result in varying degrees of whole-network improvement (Figure 4.16 to Figure 4.23).

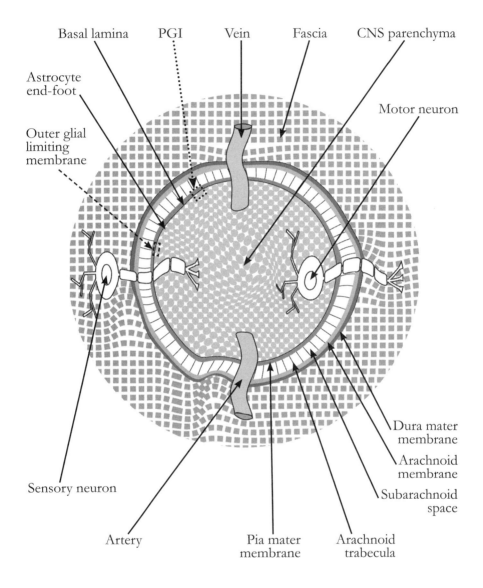

Figure 4.16. Diagram of fascial-glial network strain. Fascial strain distorting nerves, vessels, and the PGI. The PGI transfers the fascial patterns into the CNS parenchyma.

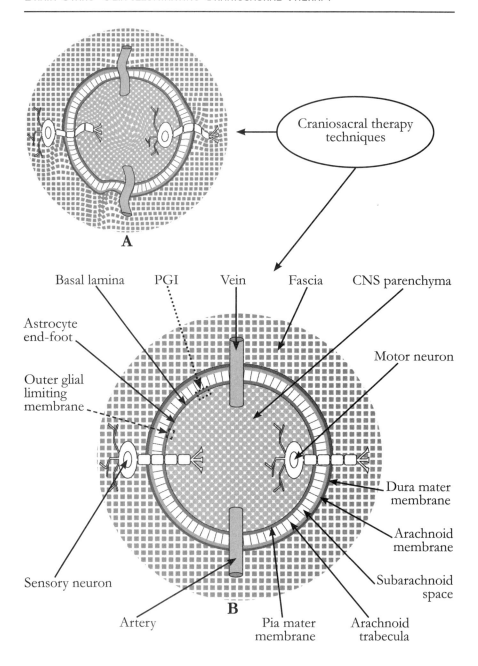

Figure 4.17. Diagram of fascial-glial strain correction. **A:** Fascial strain distorting nerves, vessels, PGI, and CNS parenchyma. **B:** Craniosacral therapy techniques can facilitate correction of strain patterns, which lessens adverse structural stress that can lead to functional correction.

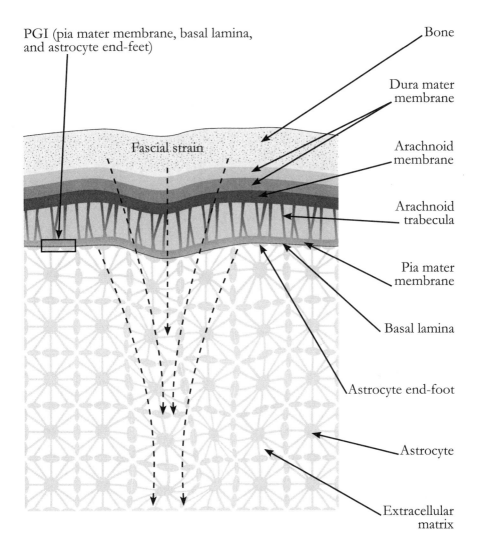

Figure 4.18. Fascial strain transmitted into the PGI, glial syncytium, and extracellular matrix in such a way that the brain tissue is compressed or twisted.

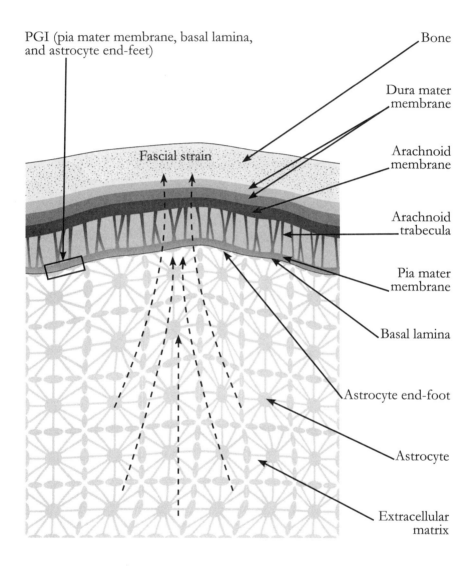

Figure 4.19. Fascial strain transmitted into the PGI, glial syncytium, and extracellular matrix in such a way that the brain tissue is pulled towards the fascial strain.

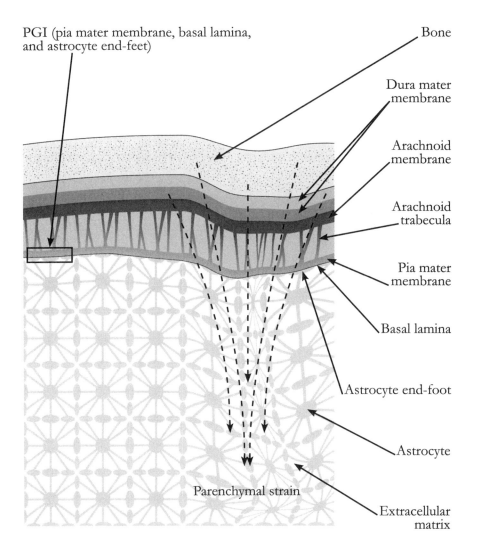

Figure 4.20. Parenchymal strain transmitted through the glial syncytium and extracellular matrix to the PGI. The PGI transmits strain in such a way that the surrounding fascia is pulled into the parenchymal strain.

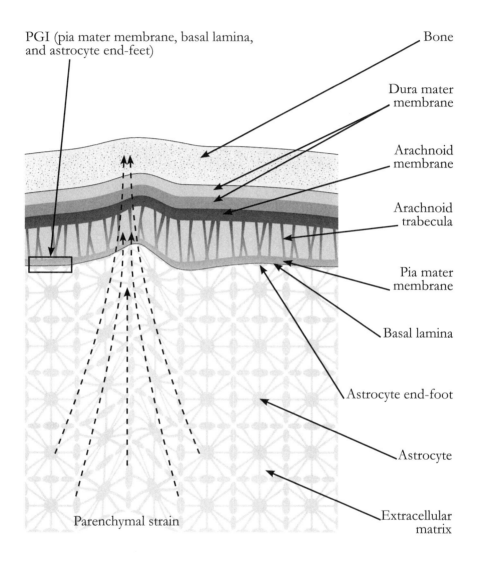

Figure 4.21. Parenchymal strain transmitted through the glial syncytium and extracellular matrix to the PGI. The PGI transmits strain in such a way that the surrounding fascia is pushed outward and is deformed.

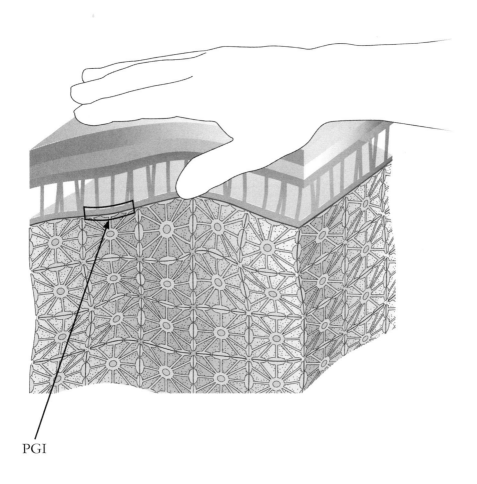

PGI

Figure 4.22. Feeling biomechanical adverse strain patterns though the PGI.

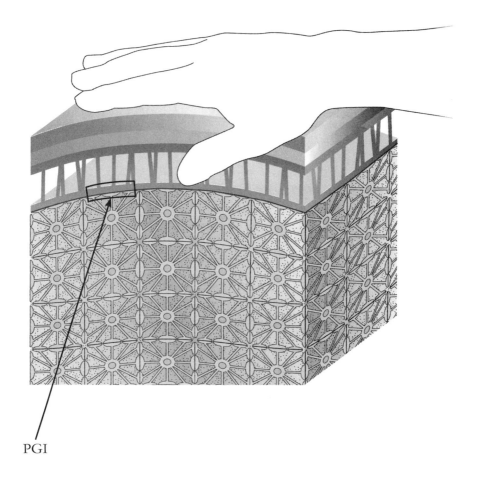

Figure 4.23. Facilitating correction of biomechanical adverse strain patterns. through the PGI.

Chapter 5

Cerebrospinal fluid and its glial connection

Glial cells are vital in all aspects of cerebrospinal fluid (CSF) physiology because they:
- produce CSF,
- form channels through which CSF flows, and
- regulate the circulation of CSF into and out of the CNS parenchyma.

CSF circulation is called the body's "third circulatory system" because it is essential to overall health and function. The other two circulatory systems are the "cardiovascular" and "lymphatic."

In this chapter we will discuss CSF in the following sections:
- the importance of CSF,
- CSF production sites,
- glial regulation of CSF circulation,
- interstitial fluid,
- CSF reabsorption sites, and
- craniosacral system and CSF dynamics.

The importance of CSF

CSF appears during the fourth week of embryonic development within an area of the developing CNS called the "lumen of the neural tube." The lumen (opening) of the neural tube will become the ventricular system. CSF is essential for typical development of the embryonic and fetal CNS.

The neural tube lumen is lined with a layer of stem cells called "germinal neuroepithelial cells." This cell layer is called the "ventricular zone" (Figure 5.1). Along the outer surface of the ventricular zone (the side facing towards the developing CNS) is another stem cell area called the "subventricular zone" (Figure 5.1). Both zones contain stem cells that generate CNS neurons and glia.

Recent research shows that the subventricular zone persists along an area of the lateral ventricles throughout life (Figure 5.2). Astrocytes within this zone have stem cell-like properties capable of generating new neurons and glia. These astrocytes extend a thin hairlike extension of their cell body into the ventricular cavity to remain in direct contact with ventricular CSF. Although the purpose of this CSF contact has not been defined, it may be essential in supporting the survival and function of these stem cell-like astrocytes.

CSF growth factors

CSF contains substances called "growth factors" and "vitalizing (trophic) factors." These factors nourish and stimulate stem cells in both the ventricular zone and subventricular zone and enable the development of neurons and glia. These CSF substances also nourish, stimulate, and support the growth of the developing neurons and glia.

CSF growth factors are involved in the guidance of developing axons. In this regard, CSF helps regulate the architecture of the developing brain and spinal cord.

CSF pressure during development

CSF pressure within the lumen and the ventricular system during development appears to support the brain so that it does not collapse inward upon itself as it grows rapidly. The brain grows by 100,000 times in volume during embryogenesis (first eight weeks of development). Equally astonishing is that approximately 2,500 new neurons are generated within the brain every minute between the second and third trimesters of fetal development.

CSF pressure generates tension into the ventricular zone, subventricular zone, and developing parenchyma, which is one way typical cell differentiation is stimulated.

After birth (postnatally) and throughout life, CSF circulates into the parenchyma carrying essential substances such as: nutrients, water, growth factors, proteins, ions, neuroendocrine substances, neuroregulators, and amino acids. These substances play a fundamental role in controlling the regulatory (homeostatic), hormonal, signaling, and repair processes within the CNS.

CSF floats the brain

CSF protects the brain by "floating" it within fluid (Figure 5.3), which reduces its effective weight in an adult from about 1400 grams (about 3 pounds) to less than 50 grams (approximately 1/10 pound). This guards the brain's blood vessels and delicate tissue from being smashed and damaged by its own weight against its bony container. CSF also protects the brain from impact as well as from sudden starts and stops.

Throughout life, CSF circulation continually cleanses the parenchyma of harmful substances. This constant cleansing is essential because the buildup of substances such as waste, toxins, or irritants can lead to parenchymal stress and eventually pathology, such as neurodegeneration. Also, poor or obstructed CSF circulation can cause hydrocephalus or cerebral hypertension.

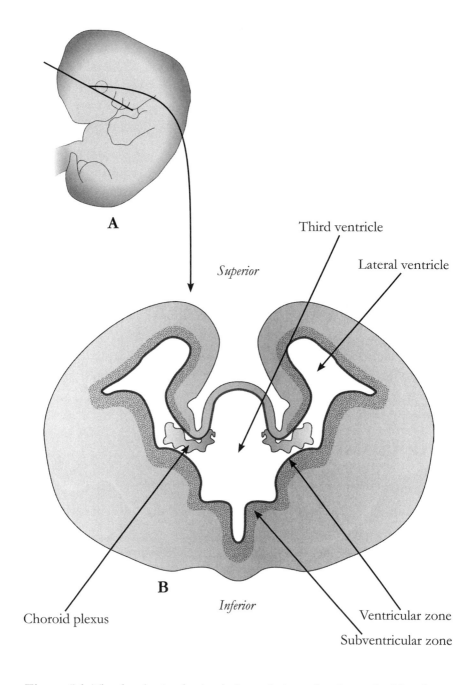

Figure 5.1. The developing brain. **A:** Lateral view of a six-week-old embryo. **B:** Coronal section of the developing embryonic brain (superior view).

CHAPTER 5   CEREBROSPINAL FLUID AND ITS GLIAL CONNECTION

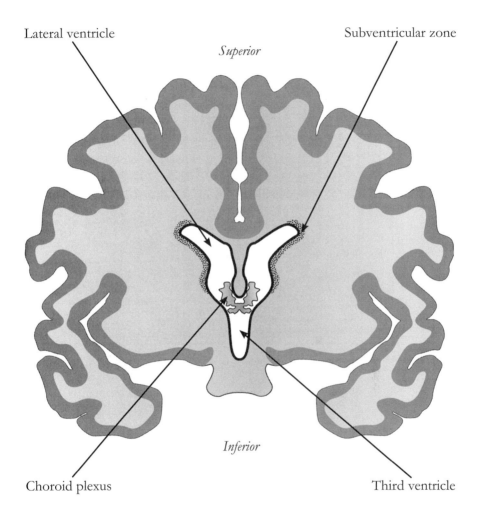

Figure 5.2. Coronal section of an adult brain (anterior view).

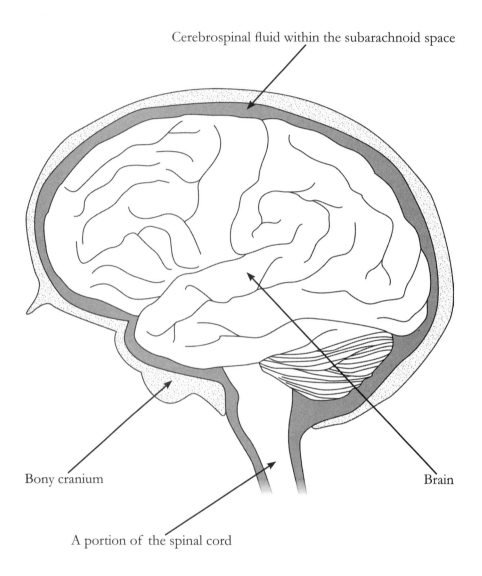

Figure 5.3. Left lateral view of the brain within the bony cranium.

CSF production sites

In the classical model of CSF physiology it is believed that the total amount of CSF is continuously produced in the ventricular system by the choroid plexuses, is absorbed into the parenchyma, and then is reabsorbed into the cardiovascular system by traveling through arachnoid villi into the dural venous sinus system. Researchers have proposed additional sites of both CSF production and reabsorption that broaden the classical model. Those that seem most relevant and are often cited in current CSF research will now be discussed using a CSF model in which the choroid plexuses are the primary, rather than the total, site of CSF production.

Two-thirds of the total volume of CSF is created by the "choroid plexuses" of the ventricular system. Additional amounts are produced by glial cells of the ventricular walls (ependymal cells), by the arachnoid membrane, and by capillaries within perivascular spaces throughout the CNS.

The total average amount of CSF of an adult is 150 milliliters (approximately two-thirds of a cup); 125 milliliters are found within the cranial and spinal subarachnoid spaces and 25 milliliters within the ventricles. The total amount of CSF is normally replenished four to five times a day. CSF production and drainage naturally decreases as a person ages.

Ventricular system CSF

CSF is produced in four interconnected cavities within the brain, called the "ventricular system" (Figure 5.4). The ventricular system cavities are lined with glia, called "ependymal cells." These cells cover the inner surface of the ventricles including the foramina (foramina of Monro) and channel (cerebral aqueduct) that interconnect the cavities. Ependymal cells also line the central canal.

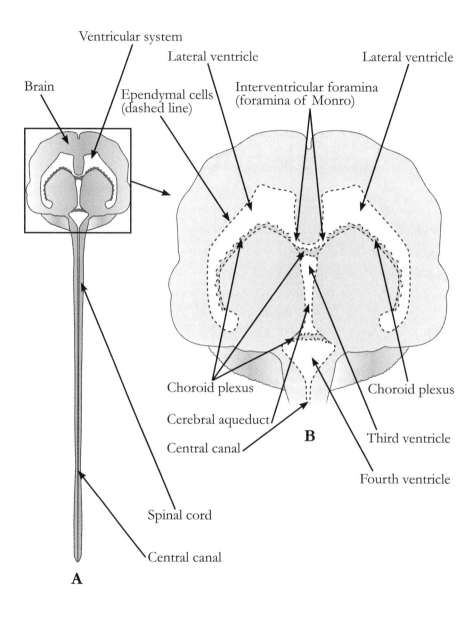

Figure 5.4. Ventricular system. **A:** Coronal section showing the brain, spinal cord, and ventricular system (anterior view). **B:** Coronal section detail of the ventricular system (anterior view).

Four ventricles

There are two ventricles lateral to the mid-line that are called "lateral ventricles," and there are two ventricles oriented along the mid-line, which are called the "third ventricle" and "fourth ventricle." The lower (inferior) aspect of the fourth ventricle extends downward (caudally) within the center of the spinal cord. This extension is shaped like a small tube and it is called the "central canal." The central canal extends from the fourth ventricle to the end of the spinal cord, which in an adult ends between vertebral levels L1-L2.

The ependymal cell surface on the inside of the ventricles is covered with tiny folds called "microvilli" and "cilia." Microvilli increase the surface area of the ventricles and absorb CSF. Cilia, which are minuscule hairlike projections of the cell, rapidly move back and forth. This motion helps circulate CSF throughout the ventricles and aids removal of debris from the cell surface. A thin layer of connective tissue called the "basal lamina" is adhered to the surface of the ependymal cells facing towards the interstitium. Astrocyte end-feet of the inner glial limiting membrane attach to the ependymal basal lamina (Figure 5.5).

Choroid plexus CSF production

CSF is produced in four separate areas, one within each ventricle, where ependymal cells surround "fenestrated capillaries." Fenestrated capillaries have small hole-like openings within their cell membrane that allow the free passage (diffusion) of blood plasma into the surrounding perivascular space. The combination of fenestrated capillaries and ependymal cells is called a "choroid plexus."

Choroid plexus capillaries are completely encased within ependymal cells (Figure 5.6). The only substances allowed entry into the ventricles are regulated by ependymal cells. The term "blood-CSF barrier" is used to refer to the combination of choroid plexus capillaries and ependymal cells. The other fluid barrier in the CNS is called the "blood-brain barrier," which is discussed in Chapter 10, "The blood-brain barrier and the neurovascular unit."

CSF is produced in two stages (Figure 5.7).

- capillary cells allow blood plasma (blood fluid without red or white blood cells) to enter the surrounding perivascular space, and
- elements from blood plasma either travel through choroid plexus ependymal cell membrane channels or they are actively transported by transmembrane proteins into the choroid plexus ependymal cells.

Once inside the cells, the substances are processed and then secreted as CSF into the ventricular cavity.

Choroid plexus CSF reabsorption

In addition to secreting CSF, choroid plexus ependymal cells also cleanse ventricular CSF of waste from cellular metabolism (metabolites), or modify CSF composition by removing excess substances, such as hydrogen or potassium. The ependymal cells are constantly cleansing CSF by reabsorbing approximately 10 percent of ventricular CSF volume (Figure 5.8).

Selective CSF substances within the ventricles travel into choroid plexus ependymal cells by either flowing through cell membrane channels, or by being transported by specialized transmembrane proteins. Once the intra-ventricular CSF substances are inside the ependymal cells they travel within the cell toward the choroid plexus perivascular space. The substances then pass into the perivascular space by traveling through membrane channels or they are actively transported by transmembrane proteins. From the perivascular space these substances are carried away by either perivascular flow or by the venous system.

CHAPTER 5 CEREBROSPINAL FLUID AND ITS GLIAL CONNECTION

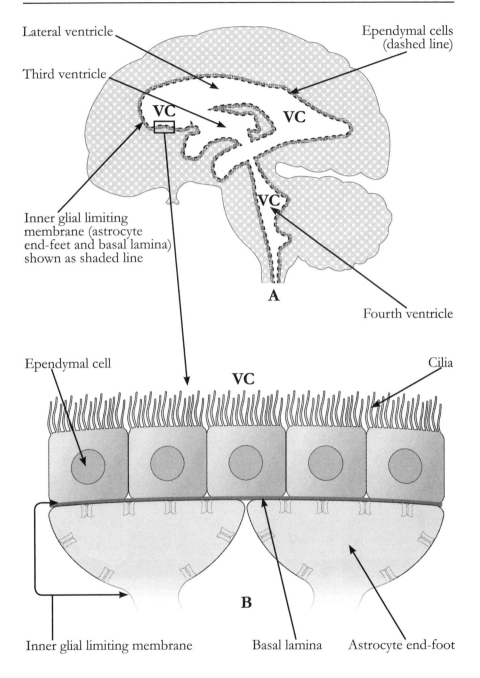

Figure 5.5. Ependymal cells. **A:** Lateral view of the ventricles. **B:** Detail of ependymal cells and the inner glial limiting membrane. "**VC**" identifies the ventricular cavity.

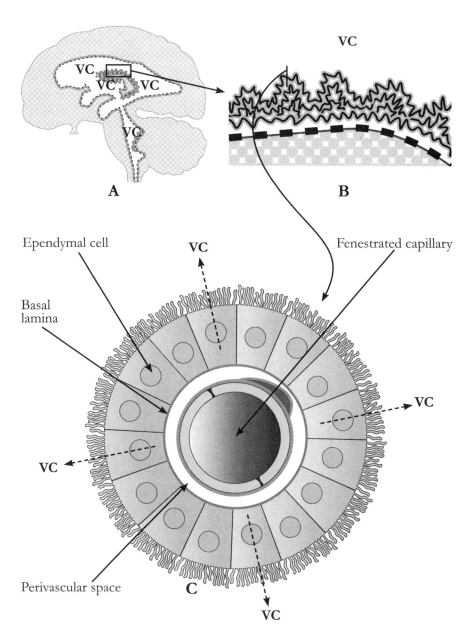

Figure 5.6. Choroid plexus. **A:** Lateral view of ventricles, choroid plexuses, and ventricular cavity (**VC**). **B:** Choroid plexus detail. **C:** Choroid plexus cross section detail. Dashed arrows show the direction of flow from a capillary into the **VC**.

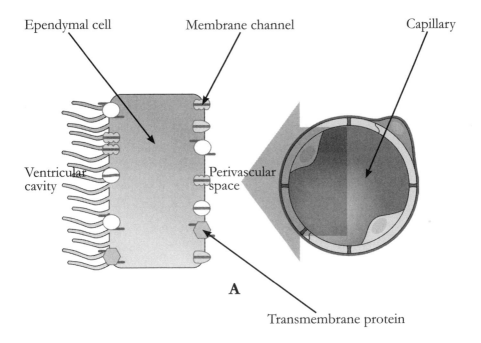
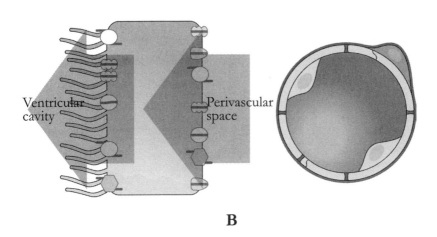

Figure 5.7. Detail of CSF production by the choroid plexus. **A:** Blood plasma flows into the perivascular space. **B:** CSF produced by ependymal cells is secreted into the ventricular cavity. Large arrows show direction of flow.

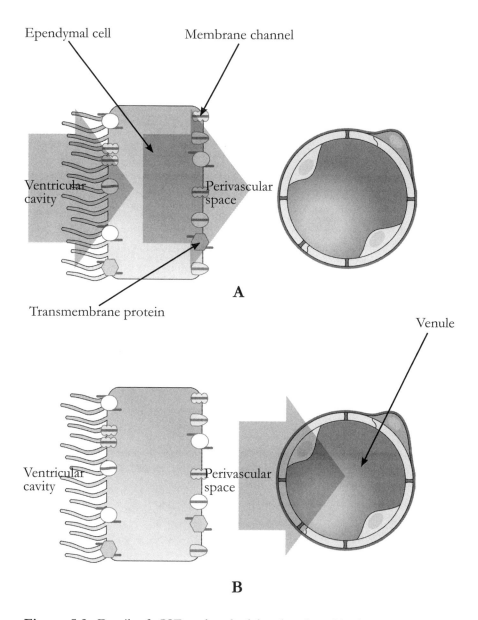

Figure 5.8. Detail of CSF reabsorbed by the choroid plexus ependymal cells. **A:** CSF reabsorbed by choroid plexus ependymal cells flows into the perivascular space. **B:** Perivascular CSF flows along perivascular pathways or enters venous capillaries (venules). Large arrows show direction of flow into a venule.

Ventricular CSF flow into the subarachnoid space

CSF flows within the ventricles in a toward-the-feet (caudal) direction into the fourth ventricle. The fourth ventricle has three openings, called "foramina," through which CSF flows into the cranial and spinal subarachnoid spaces. Two foramina are within the lateral aspects of the fourth ventricle. They are called "foramina of Luschka." One foramen is midline within the posterior aspect of the fourth ventricle. It is called the "foramen of Magendie." CSF also flows from the fourth ventricle caudally within the central canal (Figure 5.9).

Ependymal cell CSF

Ependymal cells produce CSF through the uptake of substances from both the brain parenchyma and the vasculature nearby the ependymal cell basal surface (the surface facing towards the interstitium). Substances pass through channels within astrocyte end-feet of the inner glial limiting membrane, flow through the basal lamina, and then enter ependymal cells.

Ependymal cells use parenchymal and blood substances to produce CSF, which is secreted into the ventricles to combine with CSF produced by the choroid plexuses (Figure 5.10).

Tanycytes within the ventricular wall

Tanycytes, a form of glial cell, are found within the ependymal cell layer. They extend into the ventricular cavities to detect CSF composition and relay this information to the hypothalamus and pituitary gland, which helps to modify hormone levels. Tanycytes also seem to be able to influence cerebral blood flow and neural activity by modifying the production and release of nitric oxide within the CNS. Nitric oxide is an important chemical-signaling molecule produced in the CNS parenchyma by neurons, astrocytes, and the inner lining of CNS blood cells (endothelium).

Tanyctes also form a seal between the brain and areas in the brain that do not have a blood-brain barrier. These areas are called "circumventricular organs." The pineal gland is an example of this type of organ.

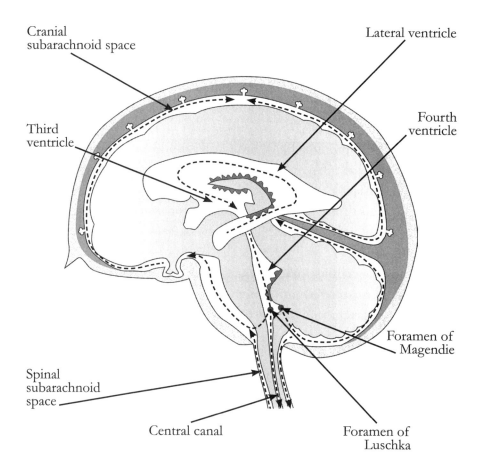

Figure 5.9. Midsagittal section showing ventricular and subarachnoid space CSF flow as dashed arrows.

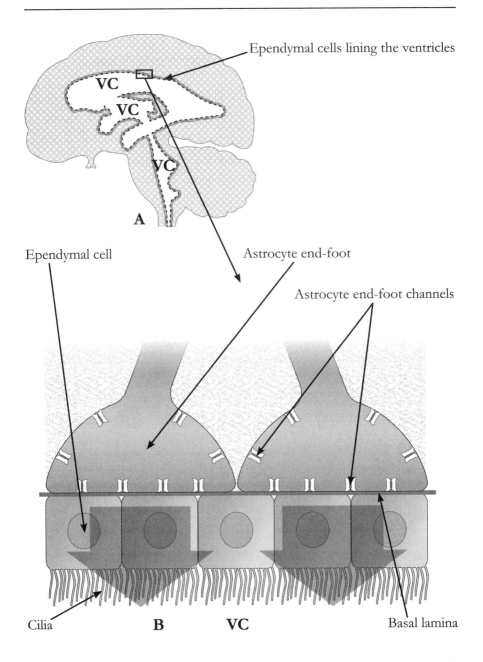

Figure 5.10. Ependymal cell CSF production. **A:** Left lateral view of ventricles. **B:** Detail of ventricular wall, astrocyte end-feet, basal lamina, and ependymal cells. Large arrows show direction of CSF flowing into the ventricular cavity. "**VC**" identifies the ventricular cavity.

Autonomic nervous system CSF regulation

The choroid plexuses receive autonomic nervous system (ANS) innervation from both the sympathetic and parasympathetic divisions. Research varies regarding ANS regulation of CSF production, such as in the following two contradictory models: 1) sympathetic innervation reduces CSF secretion, and parasympathetic innervation increases CSF secretion; 2) sympathetic innervation both increases and decreases CSF secretion, and parasympathetic innervation decreases CSF secretion. Sympathetic innervation arises from the superior cervical sympathetic ganglion. Parasympathetic innervation appears to arise from the nuclei of the vagus and glossopharyngeal nerves (Figure 5.11).

Arachnoid membrane CSF

The arachnoid membrane is one of the meningeal layers encasing the CNS. It is composed of approximately five layers of densely packed and tightly interconnected "fibroblasts," ground substance, and fibrous proteins. Fibroblasts are cells that produce the ground substance and fibrous proteins that make up connective tissue. The density of fibroblasts found within connective tissue varies throughout the body. The arachnoid membrane produces CSF that flows into the subarachnoid space (Figure 5.12).

CNS capillary CSF

Astrocyte end-feet and basal lamina surround all CNS blood vessels that are within the parenchyma (estimated at 400 miles of blood vessels). A small space exists between the outside of these blood vessels and astrocyte end-feet. This space is called a "perivascular space." At the capillary level, elements move though the blood vessel wall and then pass into the surrounding perivascular space. Some of these elements are considered CSF (Figure 5.13 and Figure 5.14).

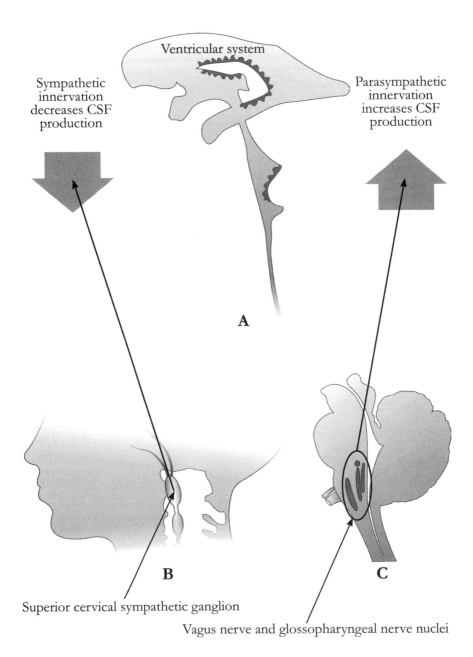

Figure 5.11. A model of autonomic nervous system regulation of CSF production. **A:** Ventricular system. **B:** Lateral view of the superior cervical sympathetic ganglion. **C:** Lateral view of the brainstem.

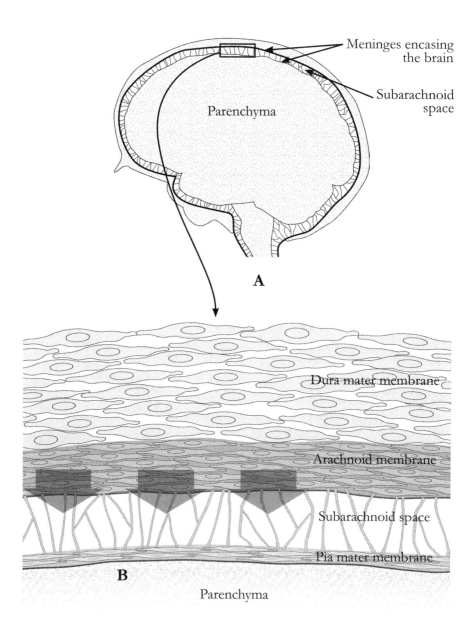

Figure 5.12. CSF produced by the arachnoid membrane. **A:** Midsagittal section of the brain. **B:** Detail of meninges. Large arrows show CSF flowing into the subarachnoid space.

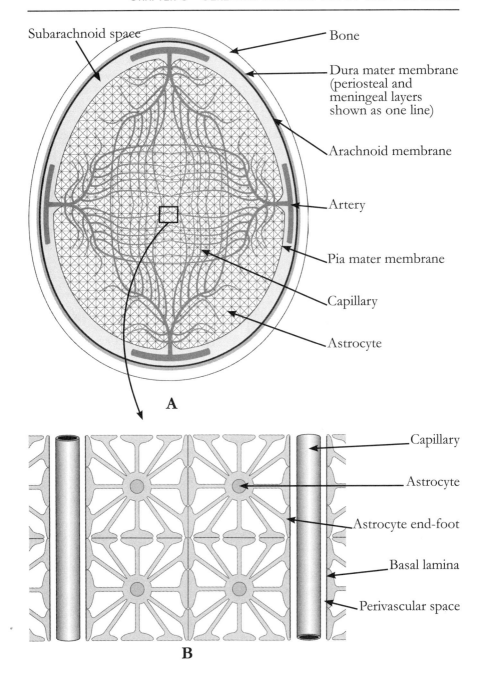

Figure 5.13. Parenchymal capillaries surrounded by astrocyte end-feet and basal lamina. **A:** Transverse section of the brain showing blood vessels and astrocyte matrix. **B:** Detail of astrocyte end-feet and capillaries.

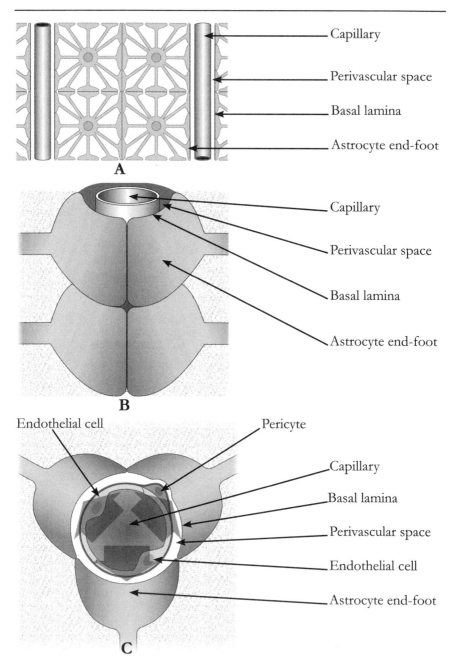

Figure 5.14. CSF capillary production. **A:** Detail of astrocytes and capillaries. **B:** Anterior detail of astrocyte end-feet encasing a capillary. **C:** Transverse section of a capillary and end-feet. Large arrows show CSF flow into the perivascular space.

Glia regulation of CSF circulation

The CNS does not have lymphatic vessels, yet it is crucial for CNS health and function that the spaces between its cells (extracellular space) and the fluid within the extracellular space (interstitial fluid) is cleansed. Research regarding how CSF flows into and out of the CNS interstitium shows that a dynamic clearance system exists throughout the CNS. This system is called the "glymphatic system."

By injecting florescent dye into the ventricular system in anesthetized mice, researchers noted that small amounts of CSF flowed through ependymal cells and then into the brain parenchyma, but CSF did not enter the subarachnoid space. (This is in contrast to the classical CSF model that proposes ventricular CSF only flows into the subarachnoid space.)

Glymphatic system CSF flow

Researchers also injected florescent dye into a large subarachnoid space of the mice, called the "cisterna magna," and found that the dye flowed quickly into the brain parenchyma. They followed the cisterna magna dye as the dye flowed within the subarachnoid space (Figure 5.15) and then:
- entered the CNS interstitium by traveling through both the pia mater membrane and the outer glial limiting membrane,
- traveled along the outside of blood vessels (arterial perivascular space),
- entered the CNS interstitium through astrocyte water channels, called "aquaporins,"
- mixed with CNS interstitial fluid,
- exited the CNS interstitium by traveling through astrocyte aquaporins,

- flowed into the space outside of blood vessels (venous perivascular space), and
- was reabsorbed through arachnoid villi into the dural venous sinus system.

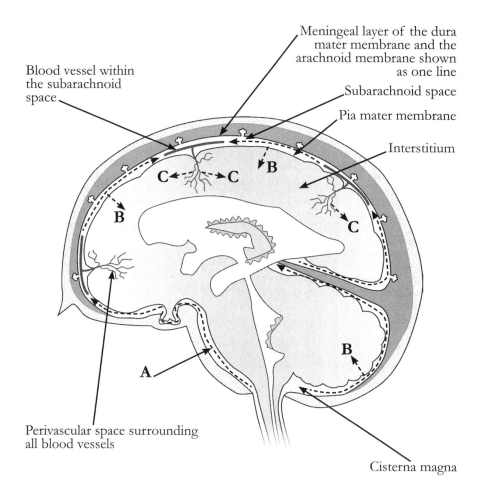

Figure 5.15. CSF flow into the interstitium. Midsagittal section of the brain. Dashed arrows show CSF flowing within the (**A**) subarachnoid space. Dashed arrows show CSF flowing into the interstitium (**B**) through the pia mater membrane and the outer glial limiting membrane and (**C**) through the perivascular glial limiting membrane.

Pia mater membrane CSF flow

CSF within the subarachnoid space flows through the pia mater membrane, through the basal lamina, and then through aquaporins within the outer glial limiting membrane to enter the interstitium (Figure 5.16).

Perivascular CSF flow

Perivascular spaces typically exist wherever blood vessels are found within the CNS parenchyma. Astrocyte end-feet forming the perivascular spaces are adhered to a connective tissue layer called the "basal lamina." The combination of perivascular astrocyte end-feet and its basal lamina layer is called the "perivascular glial limiting membrane." This membrane is a barrier regulating the flow of substances in two directions, which are from the:
- perivascular space into the interstitium, and
- interstitium into the perivascular space.

CSF produced in all four ventricles by the choroid plexuses (classical CSF model) and ependymal cells flows into the subarachnoid space to mix with CSF produced by the arachnoid membrane. This collective subarachnoid-space CSF flows into spaces around blood vessels traveling through the pia mater membrane to enter the parenchyma. These spaces are known as "Virchow-Robin" spaces (Figure 5.17). Once CSF flows through Virchow-Robin spaces it then flows along perivascular spaces formed by the perivascular glial limiting membrane.

At the capillary level, CSF flows through the perivascular glial limiting membrane basal lamina, and then flows through channels in the astrocyte end-feet, called "aquaporins," to enter the CNS interstitium (Figure 5.18). The majority of CSF from perivascular spaces flows into the interstitium through aquaporin channels, while a small amount flows through tiny spaces in between end-feet.

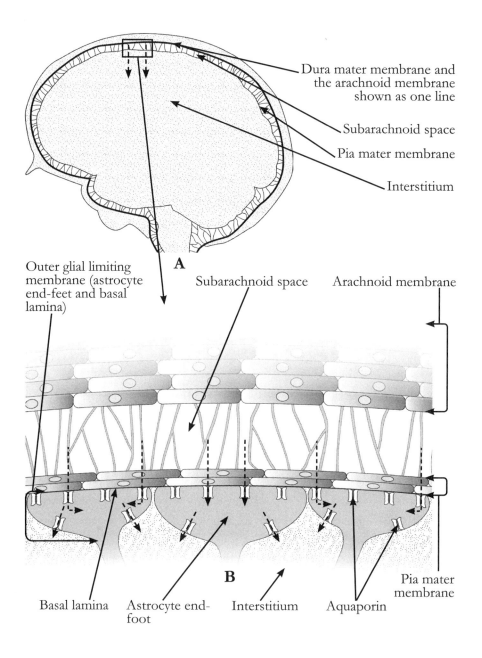

Figure 5.16. Pia mater membrane CSF flow. **A:** Midsagittal section of the brain. **B:** Detail of the pia mater membrane. The outer glial limiting membrane is also shown. Dashed arrows show CSF flow into the interstitium.

CHAPTER 5   CEREBROSPINAL FLUID AND ITS GLIAL CONNECTION

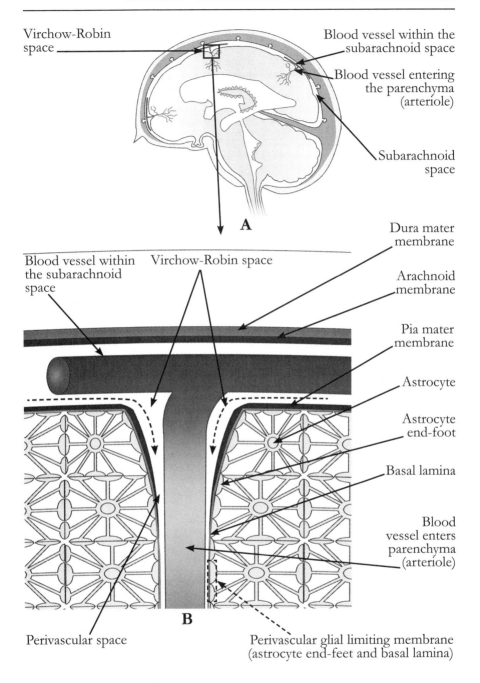

Figure 5.17. Virchow-Robin space. **A:** Midsagittal view of the brain. Blood vessels within the subarachnoid space. **B:** Virchow-Robin space detail. Dashed arrows show CSF flow into Virchow-Robin space and perivascular space.

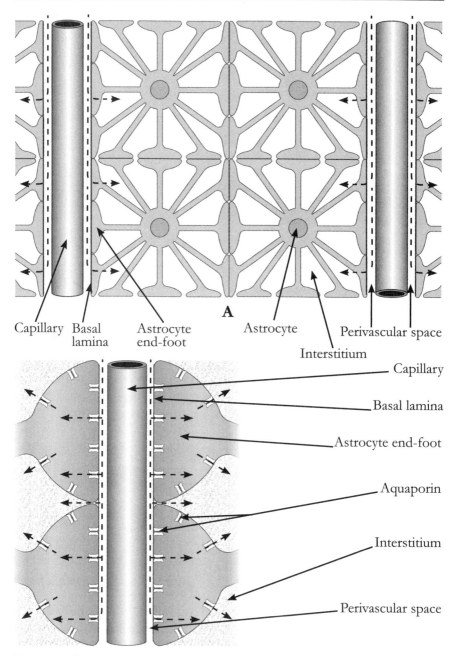

Figure 5.18. Perivascular CSF flow. **A:** Astrocyte end-feet form the perivascular space. **B:** Detail showing astrocyte end-feet, aquaporins, basal lamina, and perivascular space. Dashed arrows show CSF flow through the basal lamina, through aquaporins, and then into the interstitium.

Ependymal cell CSF flow

CSF within the ventricles flows into ependymal cells, through the basal lamina, and then through aquaporins within the inner glial limiting membrane to enter the interstitium (Figure 5.19).

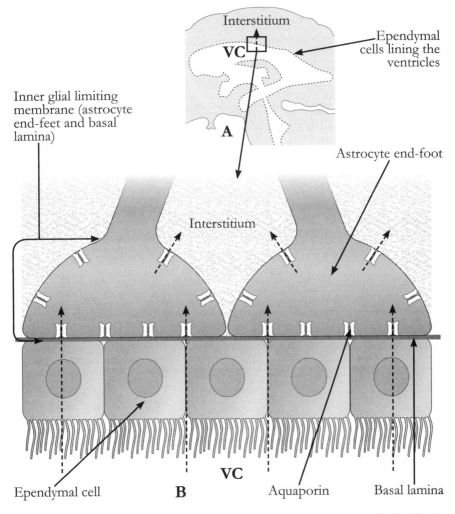

Figure 5.19. Ependymal CSF flow. **A:** Midsagittal section of the brain showing the ventricles. **B:** Detail showing astrocyte end-feet, aquaporins, basal lamina and ependymal cells. Dashed arrows show CSF flow into the interstitium. "**VC**" identifies the ventricular cavity.

Interstitial fluid

When CSF and elements from blood enter the interstitium they combine to be called "interstitial fluid" (ISF). ISF and CSF have almost the identical water content, which is 98.5 percent for ISF and 99 percent for CSF. In essence, all substances moving throughout the interstitium are carried by water. Unobstructed and efficient movement of ISF supplies CNS cells with essential fluid and critical ISF substances that allow the brain and spinal cord to function. ISF circulation also helps flush debris, toxins, and inflammatory molecules out of the interstitium, which is crucial because buildup of these substances can lead to debilitating disorders like Parkinson's disease, Alzheimer's disease, dementia, epilepsy, or depression.

CSF reabsorption pathways

As discussed earlier, glymphatic system researchers found that florescent dye injected into a large subarachnoid space (cisterna magna) of mice flowed into the interstitium through perivascular glial limiting membrane aquaporins and mixed with interstitial fluid.

The researchers also found that florescent dye flowed out of the interstitium by traveling through perivascular glial limiting membrane aquaporins. In their research, the florescent dye was then reabsorbed into the dural venous sinus system primarily by flowing into the straight sinus and transverse sinuses.

The proposed amount of CSF reabsorbed through various pathways differs among researchers. Three are listed below:
- 95 percent through cranial arachnoid villi into the dural venous sinus system;
- 50 percent through olfactory perineural channels, 25 percent through cranial arachnoid villi, 25 percent through spinal arachnoid villi; and

- almost all CSF is reabsorbed into the circulatory system by draining into venous capillaries (venules).

The full range of CSF drainage routes and reabsorption pathways known to date are described below. CSF must exit the CNS interstitium before it can be reabsorbed into the circulatory and lymphatic systems. CSF exits the interstitium by flowing through the:
- outer glial limiting membrane and pia mater membrane, or;
- perivascular glial limiting membrane.

CSF passing through the outer glial limiting membrane will flow through the pia mater membrane, and then flow into the subarachnoid space. CSF passing through the perivascular glial limiting membrane will flow into the perivascular space. Once CSF has flowed into the subarachnoid space or the perivascular space, it will be reabsorbed into either the vascular system or the lymphatic system through the following pathways (Figure 5.20):
- cranial arachnoid villi,
- perineural spaces,
- venules,
- cerebrovascular basement membrane, and
- spinal arachnoid villi.

Outer glial limiting membrane and pia mater membrane CSF flow

CSF exits the interstitium by flowing through aquaporins within astrocyte end-feet of the outer glial limiting membrane, through the pia mater membrane and then into the subarachnoid space (Figure 5.21). This CSF will travel from the subarachnoid space, through AV, to then be reabsorbed into the circulatory system. CSF will also flow from the subarachnoid space into the lymphatic system through perineural channels.

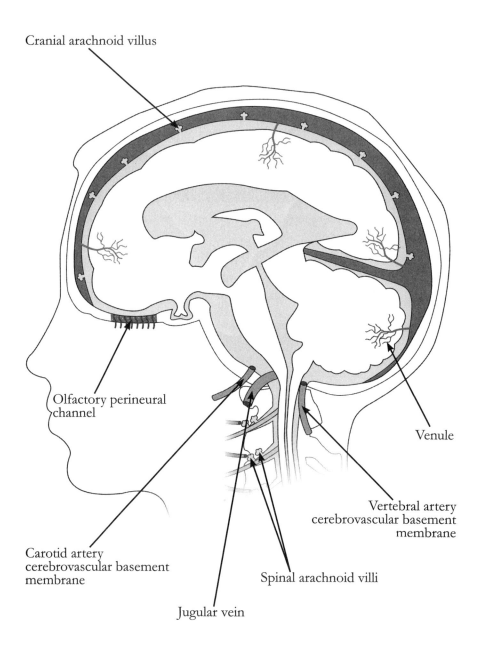

Figure 5.20. Midsagittal view showing CSF reabsorption pathways. The jugular vein is also shown.

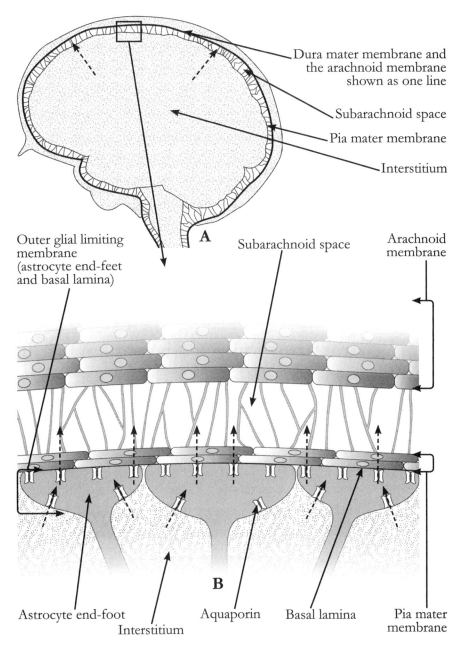

Figure 5.21. CSF exits the interstitium by flowing through the outer glial limiting membrane and pia mater. **A:** Midsagittal view of the brain. **B:** Detail showing CSF flow from the interstitium into the subarachnoid space. Dashed arrows show the direction of CSF flow.

Perivascular glial limiting membrane CSF flow

CSF exits the interstitium by flowing through aquaporins within astrocyte end-feet of the perivascular glial limiting membrane to enter the perivascular space (Figure 5.22). This CSF will travel from the perivascular space into the subarachnoid space. Subarachnoid space CSF will then be reabsorbed into the circulatory system or the lymphatic system. CSF will also flow from the perivascular space into perineural spaces, or into perivascular channels within the basement membrane of the carotid and vertebral arteries to enter the lymphatic system.

Cranial arachnoid villi CSF reabsorption pathway

Arachnoid villi (AV) are tufts of arachnoid membrane that project directly into, or are interconnected with, the dural venous sinus system (Figure 5.23). Subarachnoid space CSF flows through AV to enter the dural venous sinus system where it mixes with venous blood within the sinuses. CSF is then reabsorbed into the circulatory system by flowing through the jugular veins into the subclavian veins and onward to the heart.

Perineural space CSF reabsorption pathway

CSF drains out of the subarachnoid space through spaces around olfactory nerve fibers called "perineural spaces," passes through the cribriform plate of the ethmoid bone, and then flows into the lymphatics of the neck (Figure 5.24 and Figure 5.25). Some CSF also drains through perineural spaces of the optic nerves, trigeminal nerves, and auditory nerves.

Venule CSF reabsorption pathway

CSF passes through the perivascular glial limiting membrane, into the perivascular space, and then into venules that merge with veins. Most of the veins will interconnect with the dural venous sinuses through which CSF will be reabsorbed into the circulatory system (Figure 5.26).

Cerebrovascular basement membrane CSF reabsorption pathway

The cerebrovascular basement membrane is a thin sheet of extracellular matrix molecules covering the outer surface of blood vessels and pericytes. CSF flows through the perivascular glial limiting membrane, into the perivascular space, and then into the cerebrovascular basement membrane of capillaries. This CSF will eventually flow within the cerebrovascular basement membrane of the carotid and vertebral arteries and then into cervical lymphatics (Figure 5.27).

Spinal arachnoid villi CSF reabsorption pathway

CSF drains out of the spinal cord subarachnoid space through spinal arachnoid villi (SAV). SAV are located in two places nearby dorsal root ganglia. SAV either project into radicular veins or project into the interstitium external to the dural sac.

CSF draining through SAV into radicular veins is reabsorbed into the circulatory system. Radicular veins are small veins within the subarachnoid space located adjacent to both the dorsal and ventral roots (Figure 5.28 and Figure 5.29). Radicular veins pass through the dural sac to join the intervertebral vein.

SAV also extend from the subarachnoid space and project through the dura mater membrane to extend into the surrounding interstitium (Figure 5.29). CSF draining through these SAV merges with interstitial fluid to be reabsorbed into the lymphatic system.

Craniosacral system and CSF dynamics

CSF production sites, as well as inflow and outflow spaces, interconnect with the craniosacral system (CSS). If the CSS is distorted, even in the most minute pattern, then the distortion can alter the form of the:
- subarachnoid space,
- Virchow-Robbins spaces,
- perivascular spaces,
- perivascular glial limiting membrane,
- inner glial limiting membrane,
- outer glial limiting membrane,
- ependymal cells,
- choroid plexuses,
- aquaporin channels,
- basal lamina,
- glial matrix,
- neurons, and
- blood vessels.

Distortion of any of these structures can alter CSF production, or disrupt free and balanced flow of CSF. This can lead to a devitalized and/or toxic parenchyma.

Astrocyte end-feet create fluid barriers between the CNS parenchyma, interstitium, subarachnoid space, and all blood vessels within the pia mater membrane.

These barriers are the:
- outer glial limiting membrane,
- inner glial limiting membrane, and
- perivascular glial limiting membrane.

All of these glial membranes have aquaporin channels through which CSF flows both into and out of the interstitium.

Deformation of the following may lead to too little CSF circulating into or out of the brain or spinal cord:
- CSF production sites (choroid plexuses, ependymal cells, arachnoid membrane, capillaries):
- subarachnoid space,
- perivascular spaces,
- aquaporin channels of all glial limiting membranes (outer glial limiting membrane, inner glial limiting membrane, perivascular glial limiting membrane), and
- reabsorption sites (cranial arachnoid villi, spinal arachnoid villi, perivascular channels, perineural channels).

Alterations of form or function of the areas listed above can cause CNS distress due to:
- lack of vital substances entering either the parenchyma or the interstitium,
- fluid congestion leading to fluid stasis,
- toxicity,
- inflammation,
- glial scars,

- debris build up, and
- atypical CSF pressure.

These stressors may cause a wide array of difficulty. A partial list follows: neurodegeneration, insomnia, epilepsy, migraine, tinnitus, hydrocephalus, attention deficit disorder, lethargy, dysregulation of the autonomic nervous system, sensory processing disorder, cerebral hypertension, chronic pain, or memory loss.

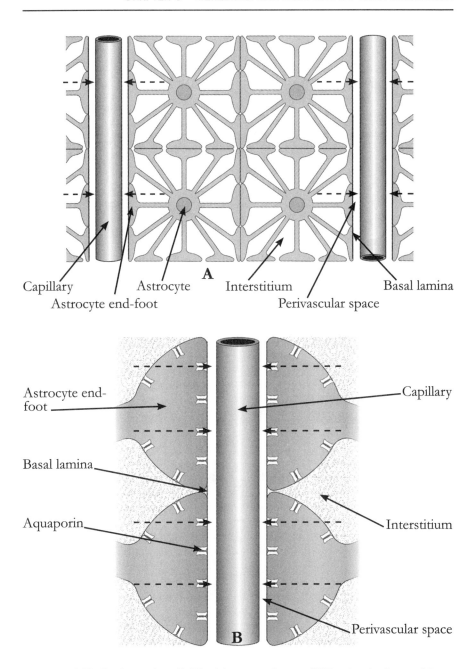

Figure 5.22. Perivascular glial limiting membrane CSF exits the interstitium. **A:** CSF flowing from the interstitium into the perivascular space. **B:** Detail showing CSF flowing through aquaporins, through the basal lamina, and into the perivascular space. Dashed arrows show direction of CSF.

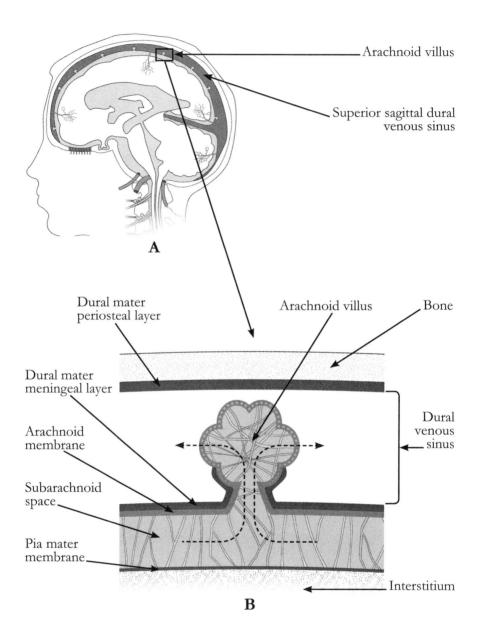

Figure 5.23. Arachnoid villi. **A:** Midsagittal view showing the superior sagittal dural venous sinus. **B:** Arachnoid villi detail. Dashed arrows show CSF reabsorption flow from the subarachnoid space into the dural venous sinus.

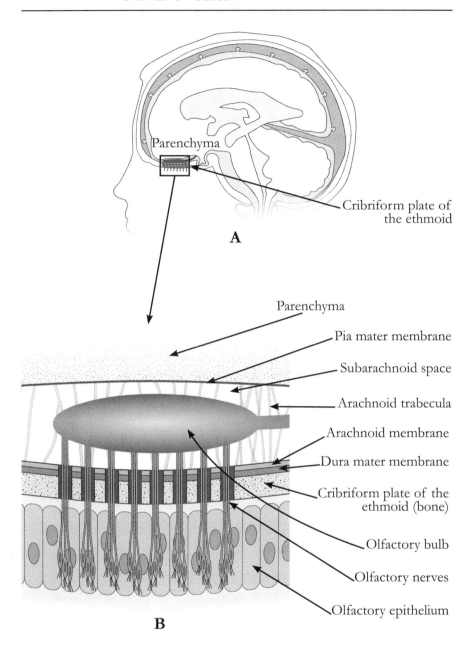

Figure 5.24. Perineural CSF drainage pathway. **A:** Midsagittal view showing the cribriform plate of the ethmoid. **B:** Lateral view detail showing olfactory nerves traveling through the cribriform plate.

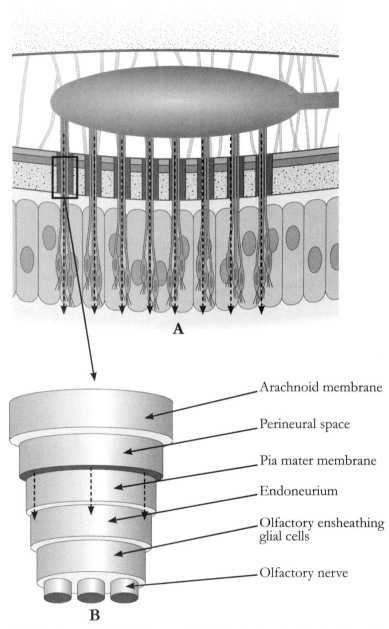

Figure 5.25. Perineural CSF drainage. **A:** Sagittal view detail showing CSF drainage within perineural channels. **B:** Lateral view detail showing olfactory nerves and perineural space. Dashed arrows show direction of CSF flowing within the perineural space.

Chapter 5 Cerebrospinal fluid and its glial connection

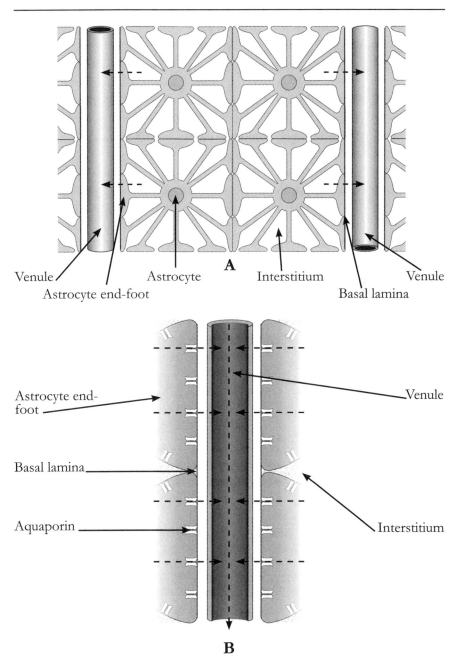

Figure 5.26. Venule CSF flow. **A:** CSF flowing from the interstitium into venules. **B:** Detail showing CSF flowing through aquaporins, through the basal lamina, and into a venule. Dashed arrows show direction of CSF.

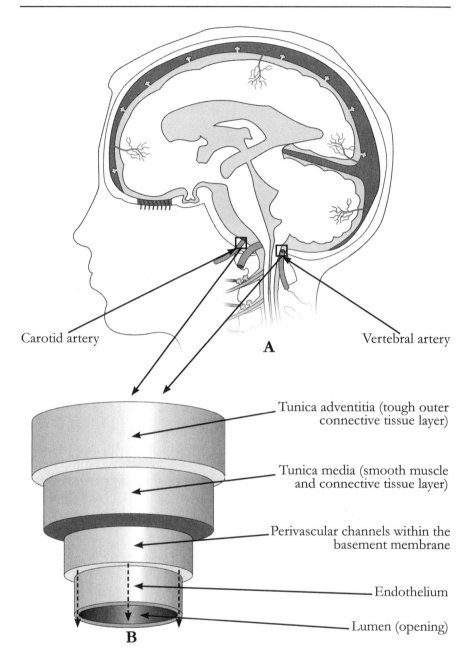

Figure 5.27. Cerebrovascular basement membrane CSF flow. **A:** Sagittal view showing the carotid and vertebral arteries. **B:** Artery detail (lateral view) showing the cerebrovascular basement membrane and connective tissue layers. Dashed arrows show CSF flowing within the cerebrovascular basement membrane.

CHAPTER 5 CEREBROSPINAL FLUID AND ITS GLIAL CONNECTION

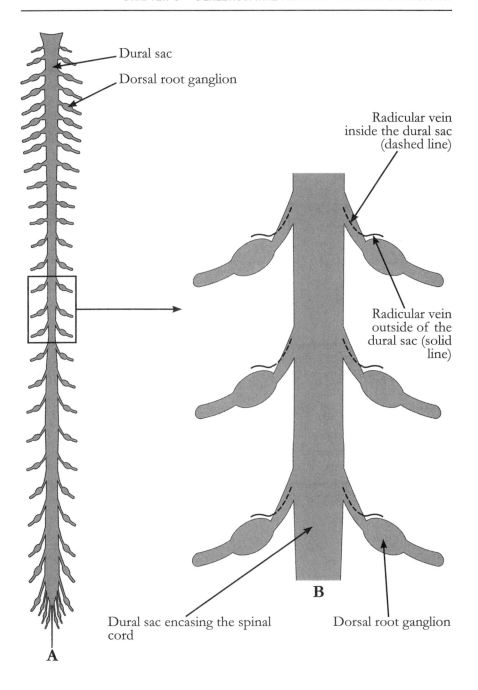

Figure 5.28. Radicular veins. **A:** Posterior view of the dural sac and dorsal root ganglia. **B:** Radicular veins inside and outside the dural sac.

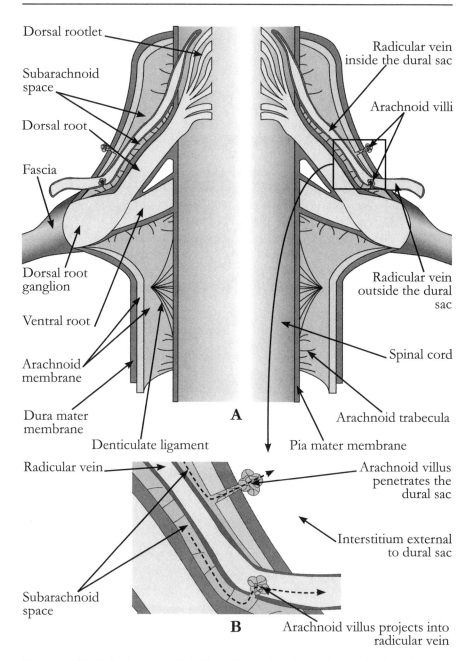

Figure 5.29. Spinal arachnoid villi. **A:** Posterior view of the spinal cord, nerve roots, arachnoid villi, and dural sac. The dural sac has been opened. **B:** Arachnoid villi detail. Dashed arrows show CSF flowing from the subarachnoid space into the interstitial fluid or into radicular vein.

Chapter 6

Radial glia and central nervous system development

Radial glia are transient glia that exist during prenatal development. This chapter has two sections:
- prenatal development stages, and
- nervous system development.

Prenatal developmental stages

There are three periods of prenatal development, which are:
- pre-embryonic,
- embryonic, and
- fetal.

Pre-embryonic period

The pre-embryonic period ranges from conception to the end of week two (Figure 6.1). During this period, the fertilized ovum moves through the uterine tube to enter the uterus. Once inside the uterus the ovum adheres to the uterine wall (implantation).

Embryonic period

The embryonic period ranges from the beginning of week three to the end of week eight (Figure 6.2). During this period, three germ (cell) layers are established, and cell specialization (differentiation) takes place that forms all of the organ systems. The three germ layers are the ectoderm, mesoderm, and endoderm.

The ectoderm

Ectodermal cells differentiate to become:
- brain and spinal cord,
- peripheral nervous system,
- Schwann cells,
- satellite glial cells,
- facial bones,
- arachnoid membrane,
- pia mater membrane,
- sensory epithelia of the eye,
- ear,
- nose,
- skin,
- nails,
- hair,
- mammary glands,
- pituitary gland,
- sweat glands, and
- enamel of the teeth.

The mesoderm

Mesodermal cells differentiate to become:
- connective tissue,
- dura mater membrane,
- cartilage,
- bone,
- striated and smooth muscle,
- blood,
- lymph vessels,
- kidneys,
- ovaries or testes,
- serous membranes lining the body cavities,
- spleen, and
- adrenal cortices.

The endoderm

Endodermal cells differentiate to become:
- gastrointestinal tract,
- respiratory tract,
- tonsils,
- liver,
- thymus,
- thyroid,
- parathyroids,
- pancreas,
- epithelial lining of the urinary bladder and urethra,
- epithelial lining of the tympanic cavity,
- tympanic antrum, and
- auditory tube.

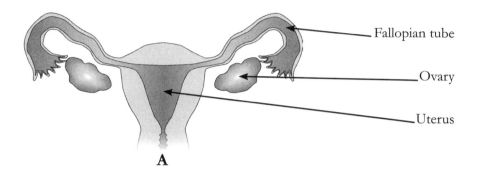

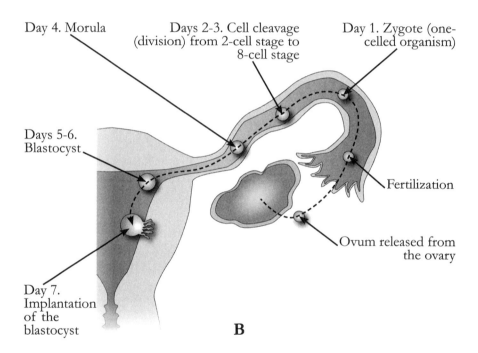

Figure 6.1. Pre-embryonic period. **A:** Anterior view of the uterus, fallopian tubes, and ovaries. **B:** Enlarged view of the left aspect of the uterus, fallopian tube, and ovary. The ovum is fertilized in the fallopian tube and travels toward the uterus. The ovum's cells increase to become a solid sphere of cells called a "morula." As the morula enters the uterus, cavities appear within its cell mass. At this stage the embryo is known as a "blastocyst." The blastocyst implants into the uterine wall.

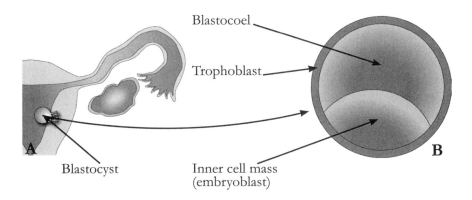
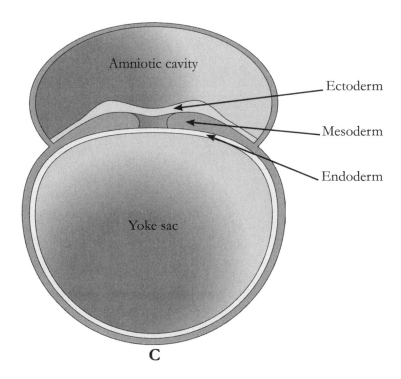

Figure 6.2. Embryonic period. **A:** Detail of a portion of the left ovary and implanted blastocyst. **B:** Blastocyst. The blastocoel is a fluid-filled cavity, the trophoblast becomes the placenta, the embryoblast forms the embryo. **C:** Gastrula. When the three germ layers develop, the embryo is known as a "gastrula."

Fetal period

The fetal period extends from the beginning of week nine to full term (38 weeks) (Figure 6.3). It is a phase of growth, development, and enlargement.

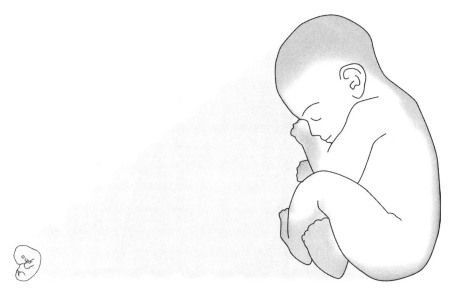

Figure 6.3. Fetal growth.

Nervous system development

The nervous system begins developing from the ectoderm at the start of the third week (Figure 6.4).

Central nervous system neurogenesis

Neurogenesis of the brain and spinal cord is the process by which cell division converts stem cells of the nervous system, called "neuroepithelial cells," into neurons and glia. Neurogenesis occurs on the surface and inside the walls of the ventricular system.

Radial glia

A transient type of glial cell called a "radial glial cell" exists during neurogenesis. Radial glia arise from neuroepithelial cells. One end of each radial glial cell attaches to the surface of the ventricles, and the cell extends outward so that the other end attaches to the inner surface of the pia mater membrane. Radial glia are like very fine strands that create an intricate framework extending from the ventricular surface to the pia mater membrane (Figure 6.5 and Figure 6.6).

Neurons travel along radial glia

Neurons emerge from ventricular neuroepithelial cells and travel along radial glia to reach their final destinations. When sliding along the length of a glial cell the pattern of motion is called, "radial migration." Neurons traveling oblique to the glial framework can pass from one glial cell to another and this is called "tangential migration." Neurons can use one or both forms of migration to reach their final destination.

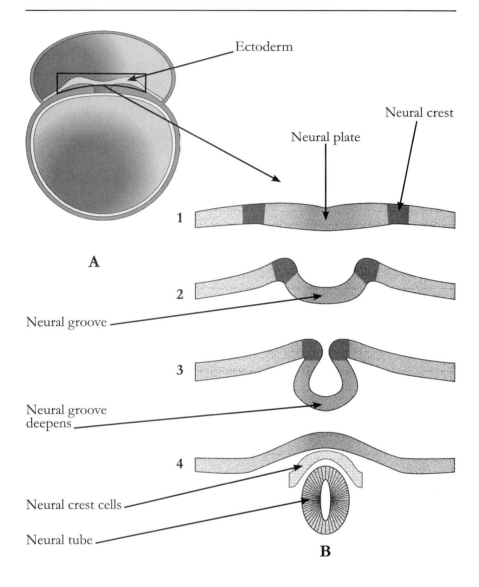

Figure 6.4. Neural tube development. **A:** Ectoderm. **B:** Neural tube formation. **1:** Between days 18-24 a portion of the ectoderm thickens into the "neural plate" and the "neural crest." **2:** The neural plate folds inward forming the "neural groove." **3:** The neural groove deepens. **4:** The neural groove detaches from the ectoderm as the "neural tube" and the neural crest detaches as a group of cells. The neural crest cells form the peripheral nervous system and a variety of other tissue. The neural tube forms the central nervous system.

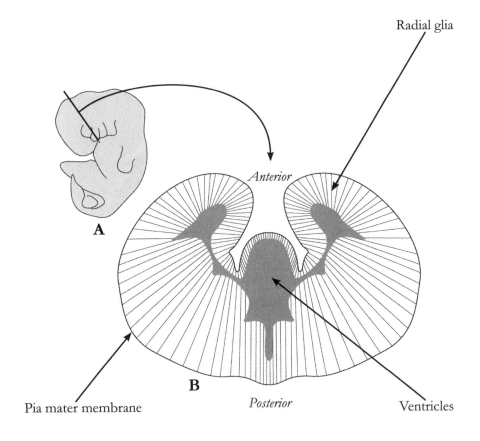

Figure 6.5. The developing brain. **A:** Line showing the direction of a transverse section through a six-week-old embryo to show the developing brain. **B:** Transverse brain section showing radial glia (superior view).

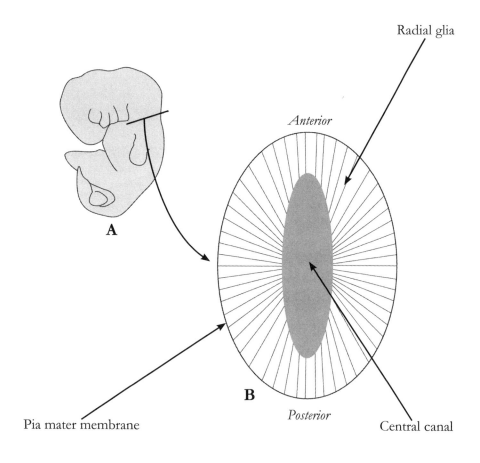

Figure 6.6. The developing spinal cord. **A:** Line showing the direction of a transverse section through a six-week-old embryo to show the developing spinal cord. **B:** Transverse section of the developing spinal cord showing radial glia (superior view).

Radial glial surface molecules help neurons find their way

Radial glial cells produce sticky or slippery molecules on their surface to help neurons find their way to their proper place within the architecture of the central nervous system (CNS). Glial surface molecules determine a neuron's final location. If the surface is sticky the neurons will continue to crawl. When they reach a slippery section they will drop off (Figure 6.7 and Figure 6.9).

Radial glial and the architecture of the CNS

Neurons traveling along radial glia suggest that radial glial may contain the overall architectural pattern of the entire CNS. Perhaps stress during this period can cause a disturbance of the glial CNS pattern, or disturb the migration of neurons, which can lead to nervous system developmental anomalies. At birth, radial glia transform into astrocytes and remain in the CNS.

Peripheral nervous system neurogenesis

The peripheral nervous system develops from neural crest cells. Neural crest cells develop from the same embryonic cell layer as the CNS, the ectodermal layer (Figure 6.4). Peripheral nervous system glia are discussed in Chapter 14, "Peripheral nervous system glia."

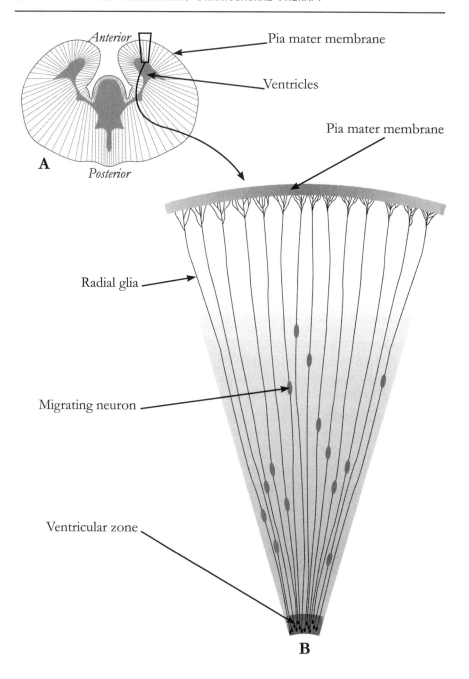

Figure 6.7. Detail of radial glia. **A:** Transverse brain section showing radial glia (superior view). **B:** Detail of radial glia. Glia and neurons arise from neuroepithelial cells of the ventricular zone (walls of the ventricles).

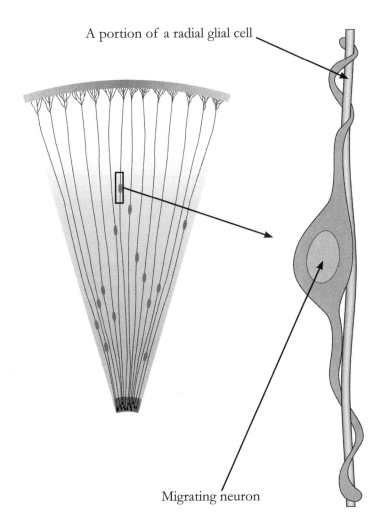

Figure 6.8. Detail of a migrating neuron.

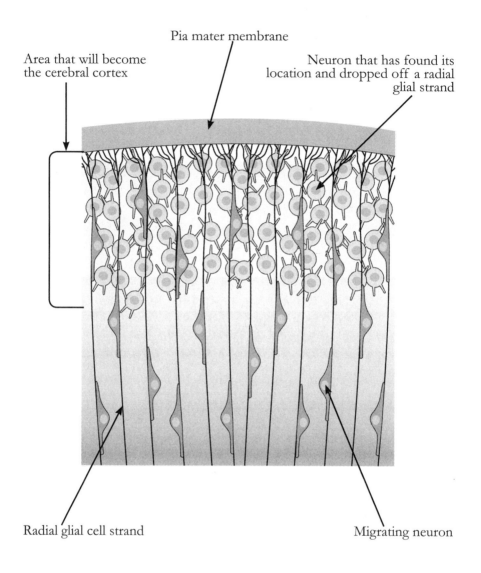

Figure 6.9. Detail of migrating neurons forming the cerebral cortex.

Chapter 7

Astrocyte overview

*A*strocytes are the most numerous and diverse glial cells in the central nervous system (CNS). They are classified into two types: "protoplasmic" astrocytes found in gray matter, and "fibrous" astrocytes found primarily in white matter (Figure 7.1).

Astrocyte cell structure

In general, each astrocyte has a central cell body with multiple processes. The end of each process expands slightly forming an "end-foot" (Figure 7.2). Within the cell body and within each end-foot are openings called "pores" or "channels" that allow for the passage of substances, such as: cerebrospinal fluid, calcium, ions, neurotransmitters, and neuromodulators (Figure 7.3).

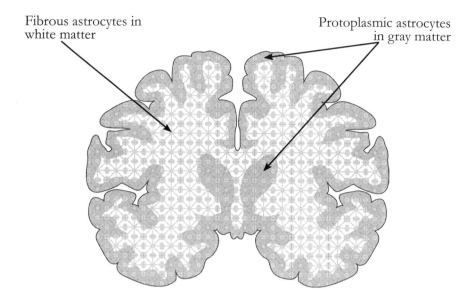

Figure 7.1. Protoplasmic and fibrous astrocytes. Anterior view of a coronal section of the brain showing gray areas as gray matter (primarily neuronal cell bodies, glia, axons, and dendrites) and white areas as white matter (predominately myelinated axons and glia).

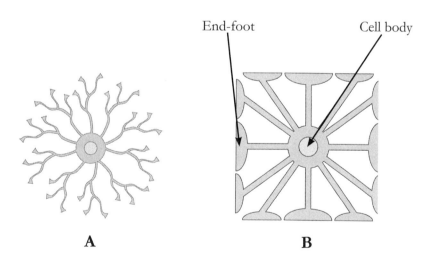

Figure 7.2. A: Simplified illustration of an astrocyte. **B:** Schematic illustration of an astrocyte.

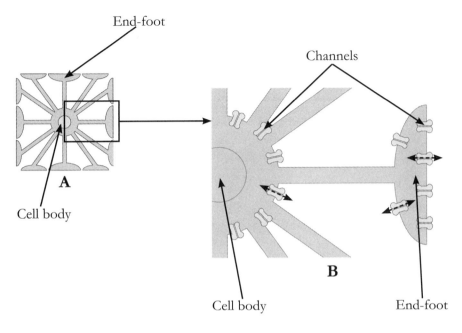
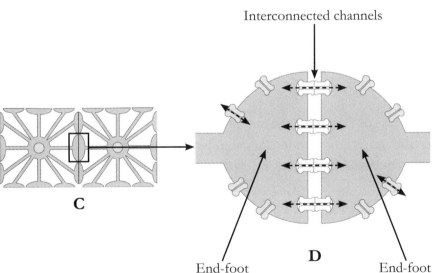

Figure 7.3. Astrocyte channel detail. **A:** An astrocyte. **B:** Enlarged portion of an astrocyte cell body and one end-foot. **C:** Two interconnected astrocytes. **D:** Interconnected channels within end-feet of two adjacent astrocytes. Dashed arrows represent the passage of substances into, out of, or between astrocytes.

Astrocytes and the glial syncytium

In the CNS, astrocyte end-feet have many interconnections. They connect with end-feet of other astrocytes and with myelin-producing glial cells, called oligodendrocytes. They also connect with the pia mater membrane and ependymal cells (cells of the ventricular system). The end-feet of astrocytes surround neurons, synapses, axons, and blood vessels.

Interconnected astrocytes (Figure 7.4) and oligodendrocytes form a matrix known as the "glial syncytium." The glial syncytium can function in many ways, such as a CNS communication network, a memory storage system, a neural network modulator, a biochemical controller, a biomechanical support and transmission network, and a CNS cleansing system. Astrocytes are the primary cells of the glial syncytium.

Glial gap junctions

Glial cells have many openings within their cell membrane, called "channels," that allow the passage of substances into and out of the cell (Figure 7.5). One of the channels is called a "gap junction" that serves as an interconnection and passageway between cells. These interconnections, formed by gap junctions, link individual glial cells into many interconnected cells that form the glial syncytium.

Glial gap junctions are formed when glia come very close together so that glial transmembrane proteins, called "connexons," align precisely to span the space between cells to form an intercellular channel (Figure 7.6). One connexon is formed by a group of six transmembrane proteins, called "connexins." Certain molecules, ions, and other substances can pass through gap junction channels. Gap junctions connect similar cells, such as astrocyte-to-astrocyte, or different cells, such as astrocyte-to-oligodendrocyte.

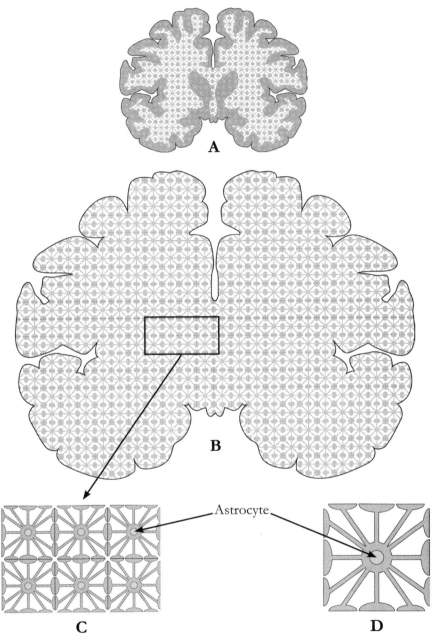

Figure 7.4. A: Coronal section of the brain (anterior view). **B:** Coronal section of the brain (anterior view) showing interconnected astrocytes of the glial syncytium. **C:** Six interconnected astrocytes. **D:** One astrocyte.

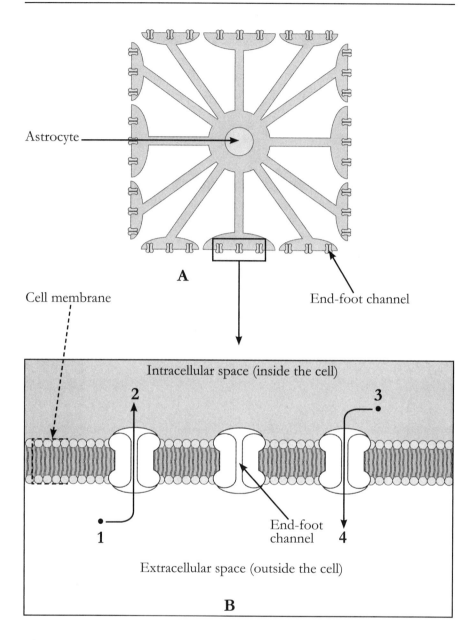

Figure 7.5. Diagram of astrocyte channels. **A:** An astrocyte showing end-foot channels. **B:** Detail of three channels in the end-foot of an astrocyte allowing for the passage of substances. **1 to 2:** Substances flow from the extracellular space into an astrocyte. **3 to 4:** Substances flow from an astrocyte's intracellular space into the extracellular space.

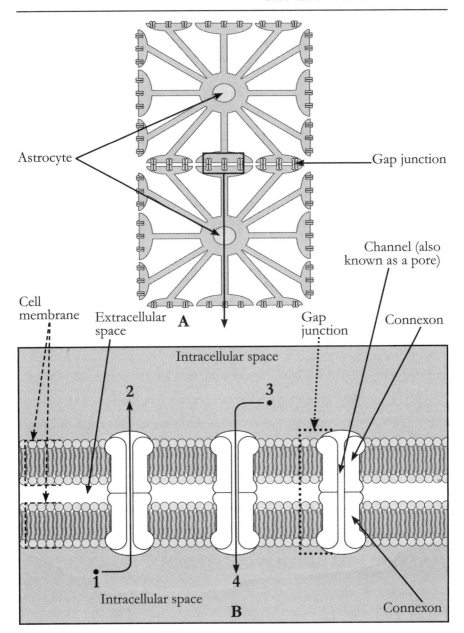

Figure 7.6. Diagram of astrocyte gap junctions. **A:** Two astrocytes showing gap junctions **B:** Detail of three gap junctions (a gap junction is formed when two connexons connect to span the extracellular space) interconnecting two end-feet allowing for the direct passage of substances between astrocytes: **1 to 2** and **3 to 4**.

Syncytial functions

The passage of intercellular substances is extremely important because it allows for glial syncytium diffusion of substances, as well as glial syncytium communication. This creates a CNS-wide system through which substances can travel far and wide to modify, integrate, and communicate with local and distant regions of the CNS (Figure 7.7). It also creates a CNS-wide information storage network. Some research suggests that memory is contained in the glial syncytium.

The glial syncytium also helps to maintain an optimal CNS environment by removing excess substances from the extracellular space, such as potassium or glutamate, in order to redistribute those substances to either areas of low concentration or to be carried away by the vascular system. This process is called "spatial buffering."

There are two types of glia that need to be free to move throughout the CNS parenchyma, they are microglia (specialized CNS immune cells) and NG-2 cells (cells with properties similar to those of stem cells). Microglia are discussed in Chapter 12, "Microglia, microgliosis, and astrogliosis."

Astrocyte mini-domains

Each astrocyte has its own separate territory where it helps to integrate the structure and function of cells with which it interconnects or surrounds (Figure 7.8). As an example, a single astrocyte may wrap about 100,000 to two million synapses. An astrocyte's mini-domain helps integrate neural signaling, control blood flow, regulate water balance, and manage many other processes in the astrocyte territory.

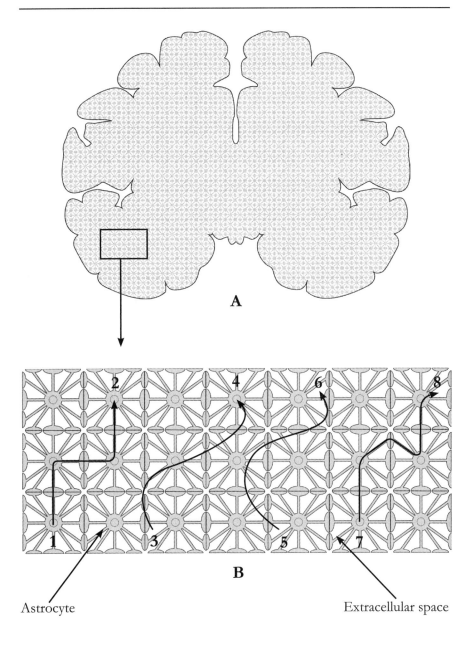

Figure 7.7. A: Coronal section of the brain (anterior view). The glial syncytium exists throughout the entire parenchyma. **B:** Detail of a portion of the astrocyte syncytium showing substances flowing. **1 to 2:** Astrocyte-to-astrocyte. **3 to 4:** Extracellular space-to-astrocyte. **5 to 6:** Extracellular space-to-extracellular space. **7 to 8:** Astrocyte to extracellular space.

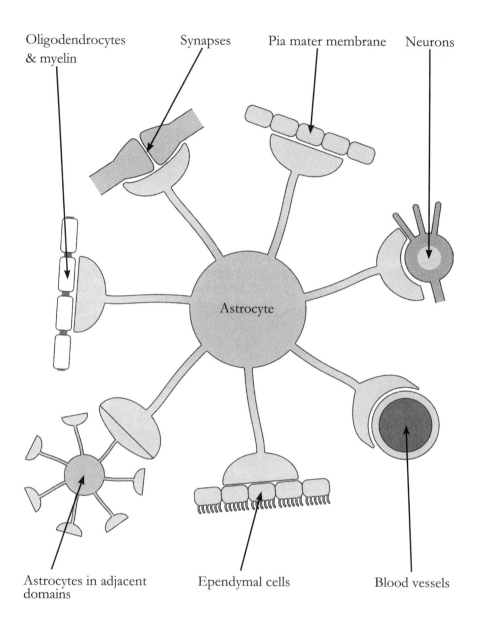

Figure 7.8. An astrocyte within its individual territory surrounds or interconnects with the structures shown above.

Astrocyte functions

Astrocytes contribute to the health and function of the CNS in innumerable ways. Some of these functions have been discussed in preceding chapters. Additional functions, such as those listed below, are described in succeeding chapters:
- regulating the concentration of substances such as neurotransmitters, neurohormones, neuromodulators, and ions within the extracellular space (ECS) that affect neural signaling;
- controlling the size and shape of the ECS, which is essential in maintaining an optimal flow of substances within the CNS;
- supplying neurons with energy (astrocytes store glucose, convert glucose to lactate, and supply lactate to neurons as needed);
- creating a CNS-wide system of syncytial communication and neural network interactions;
- controlling cerebrospinal fluid flow into and out of the CNS;
- regulating CNS water balance;
- forming part of the blood-brain barrier;
- participating in blood flow regulation;
- releasing signaling molecules called "gliotransmitters" that influence neural activity;
- modulating synaptic formation, transmission, removal ("stripping"), and networking;
- promoting myelinating activity of oligodendrocytes;
- participating in the organization of axon pathways;
- protecting and repairing the brain by producing and releasing neurotrophic substances, growth factors, and antioxidants; and
- participating in memory formation.

Chapter 8

Neurons, synapses, and astrocytes

Glial cells, in particular astrocytes, actively participate in neuronal processing, storing, and transmitting of nervous system information. Neurons communicate with other neurons through "synapses." A synapse consists of the (Figure 8.1):

- sending part of a neuron (presynaptic neuron),
- receiving part of a neuron (postsynaptic neuron), and
- minuscule gap between sending and receiving parts (synaptic cleft).

This is classically known as a "two-part synapse." The basis of two-part synaptic neuron-to-neuron interactions is the movement of either an electrical current or, most commonly, specific molecules called "neurotransmitters" through the synaptic cleft.

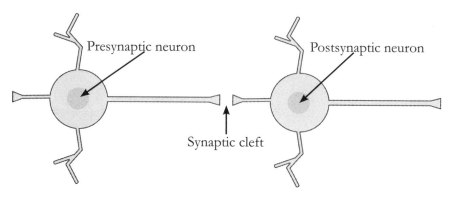

Figure. 8.1. Two-part synapse.

Synapses, numbering about 10,000 trillion in a small child and 5,000 trillion in an adult, are wrapped within astrocyte end-feet. A synapse combined with its astrocyte end-feet sheath is called a "three-part synapse" (Figure 8.2). Astrocytes help support, modify, enhance, and organize signaling at synapses.

Astrocytes and neurons are encased within the extracellular space (ECS) filled with extracellular matrix, interstitial fluid, and other substances (Figure 8.3). Molecules that help to modify and organize neural processing flow within the ECS. These substances are called "neuromodulators," and they are produced and released into the ECS by astrocytes, other glial cells, and neurons.

Neurons and the two-part synapse model

The two-part synapse model is based on "The Neuron Doctrine," which is a theory of the nervous system that has been used for over 100 years as the foundation of neuroscience and for understanding how the nervous system works.

Santiago Ramón y Cajal and Camillo Golgi shared the Nobel Prize for Physiology and Medicine in 1906 in recognition of their nervous system research. Santiago Ramón y Cajal was the main proponent of the Neuron Doctrine. Camillo Golgi was the main supporter of the "Reticular Theory" of the nervous system, in which he visualized the nervous system as a web of interconnected nerve fibers.

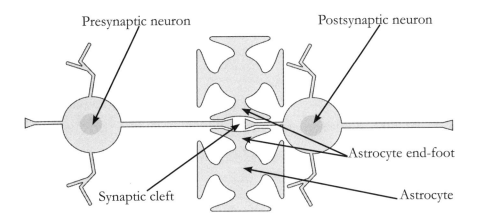

Figure. 8.2. Three-part synapse. Astrocyte end-feet encase synapse

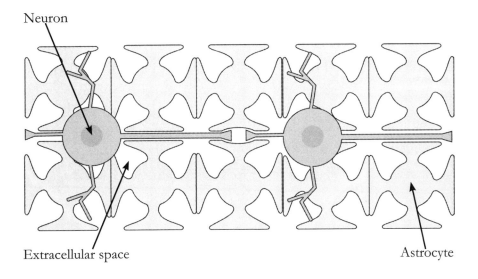

Figure. 8.3. Extracellular space surrounding both neurons and astrocytes.

Principles of the Neuron Doctrine

The Neuron Doctrine has four main principles.
- The neuron is the structural and functional unit of the nervous system.
- Neurons are individual cells that are not structurally connected to other neurons.
- The neuron has three parts: dendrites (receiving part of cell), soma (cell body), and axon (signaling part of cell) (Figure 8.4). The axon has several end branches, which make close contact to either dendrites or soma of other neurons.
- Conduction, also known as "signaling," takes place in one direction from dendrites to soma, and then on to the end of the axon branches (synapses) (Figure 8.5). Signaling occurs in very brief and very fast bursts lasting a few milliseconds.

Simple to complex information networks

In the brain there are approximately 100 billion neurons. Each of these neurons can synapse with about 10,000 other neurons. Neurons synapse with other neurons to form circuits (Figure 8.6). A few neurons synapsing with one another, called a "microcircuit," can perform tasks such as reflexes. Many microcircuits working together can create intricate networks, called "macrocircuits." Macrocircuits are involved in complex functions such as learning, memory, cognition, or artistic performance.

CHAPTER 8 NEURONS, SYNAPSES, AND ASTROCYTES

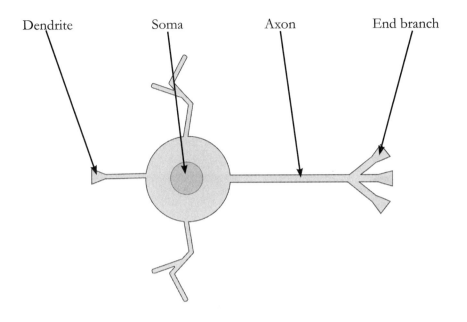

Figure. 8.4. Parts of a neuron.

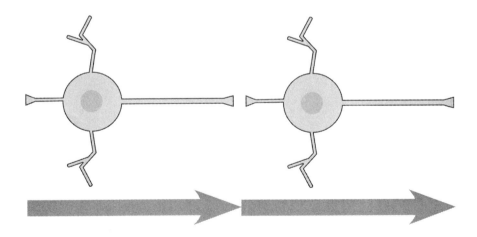

Figure 8.5. Arrows show the direction of neural conduction as described in the Neuron Doctrine.

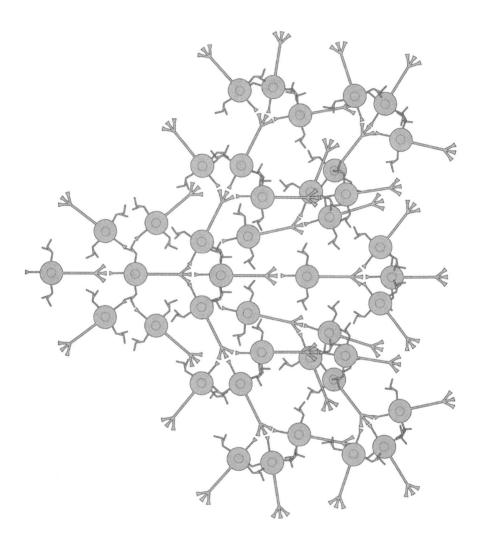

Figure 8.6. Diagram of a neural circuit.

Neuron Doctrine expanded

Recent research has revealed a number of things about neurons and glial cells that show the functional unit of the nervous system is more complex than explained by the neuron doctrine. To understand the nervous system it is helpful to use an expansion of the neuron doctrine that includes new discoveries about glial cells, neurons, and how they work together structurally and functionally.

Some new discoveries about neurons

- Neuron signaling can change spontaneously and does not always require input from other neurons.
- Some neurons form structural interconnections with other neurons or glial cells.
- Neuron signaling can last longer than milliseconds due to the effect of neuromodulatory substances, such as neuropeptides.
- Neuron signaling proceeds not only from dendrite to synapse. At times neurons have been found to signal from axon to soma or from soma to dendrites.
- Dendrites have many ion channels within their cell walls through which they receive ions from the surrounding extracellular matrix. This dendritic intake can modify dendritic reception, which regulates how a neuron responds to incoming signals from other neurons.

Some new discoveries about glial cells

- Glial cells provide neurons with essential energy substrates, especially when neurons are signaling.
- Glia help regulate and modify synaptic signaling by the uptake of neurotransmitters.

- Glia participate in the control of blood flow in tiny areas throughout the central nervous system (CNS) called "microdomains."
- Glial cells form gap junctions that interconnect glia with one another, and sometimes interconnect with neurons, into a CNS-wide matrix called a "syncytium."
- Glial cells communicate with other glia and with neurons.
- Glial gap junctions help to synchronize neuronal signaling by coupling networks into functionally interconnected micro-syncytia.
- Glial cells that create myelin in the CNS, called "oligodendrocytes," respond to neuron signaling and help support the energy demands of the neuron during signaling.
- During embryonic development, glia are the precursor cells of neurons.
- Glia and neurons form a parallel system of information processing that spread throughout the CNS over slower time scales than neural signaling.

Neurons and glia work together

The integrative workings of neurons and glia form a system of vast intricacy, flexibility, and plasticity (Figure 8.7). Current research has unveiled much about the way neurons and glia work together. This knowledge expands the Neuron Doctrine and opens new doorways in understanding the complexity and symbiotic working of neurons, glia, and the nervous system as a whole. As times goes on, increasingly more information will be discovered about the interworkings of glia and neurons that will help to open new vistas of understanding about how the nervous system works and how glial cells can be used during craniosacral therapy to lessen suffering and elevate health and healing.

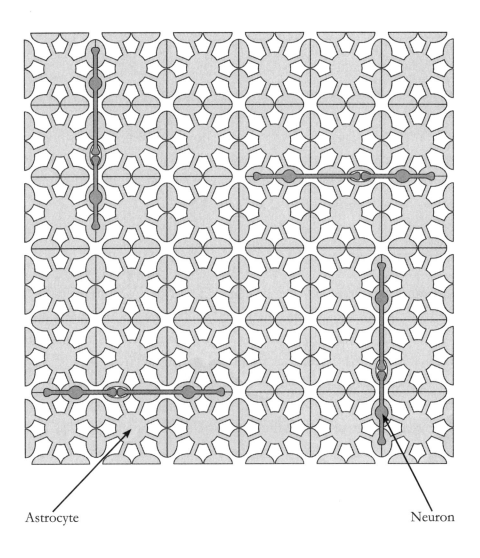

Figure. 8.7. Neurons and glia work together.

The synapse

Neurons communicate with other neurons by way of a junction called the "synapse." There are two general types of synapses: chemical synapses and electrical synapses (Figure 8.8).

Any communication between neurons occurs at a synapse. If the synapse is a chemical synapse then communication occurs within a small space between neurons called the synaptic cleft. On the other hand, when electrical currents flow between interconnected neurons, the flow takes place through channels that couple neurons together called "gap junctions." Neuronal chemical synapses are much more common than electrical synapses.

Chemical synapse

Chemical synapses are the primary means of signal transmission between neurons. This transmission takes place when chemicals, called "neurotransmitters," disperse into a minute space between sending and receiving neurons. This space is called a synaptic cleft.

A chemical synapse consists of the neuron sending a signal, called the "presynaptic" neuron, the neuron receiving the signal, called the "postsynaptic" neuron, and the synaptic cleft. The presynaptic neuron sends substances into the synaptic cleft to communicate with the postsynaptic neuron (Figure 8.9).

Neurons synthesize and then store communication molecules called "neurotransmitters" in small membrane-enclosed sacs called "vesicles." When a presynaptic neuron is activated it releases neurotransmitters from the vesicles into the synaptic cleft. Depending on the type of neurotransmitter released, the effect can either produce an excitatory response (action potential) or produce an inhibitory response in the postsynaptic neuron.

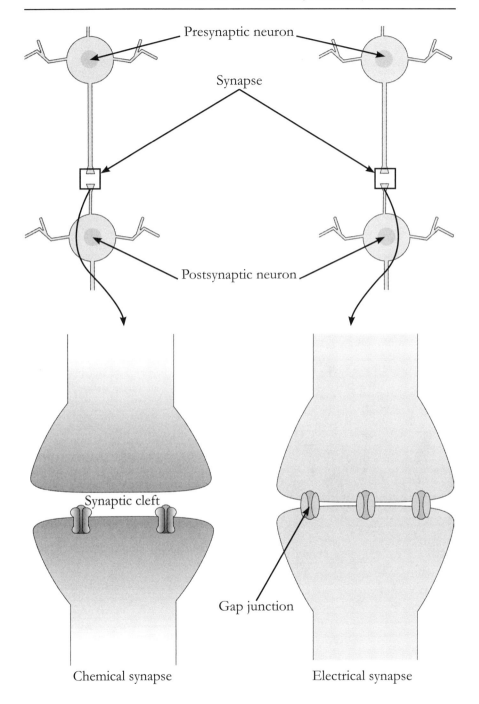

Figure 8.8. Chemical and electrical synapses.

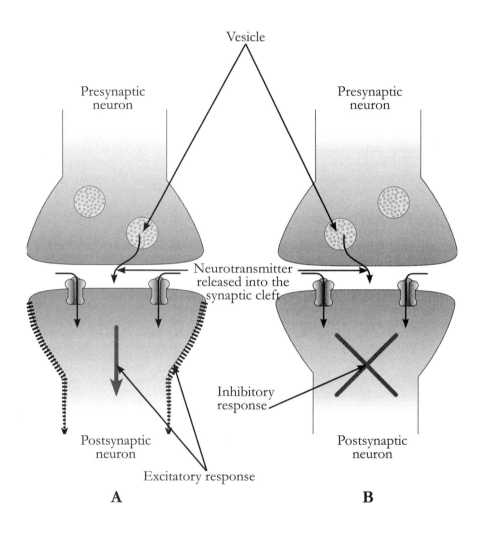

Figure 8.9. Chemical synapse neurotransmitter response. **A:** Neurotransmitter released into the synaptic cleft causes an excitatory response (action potential) in the postsynaptic neuron. **B:** Neurotransmitter released into the synaptic cleft causes an inhibitory response in the postsynaptic neuron.

Neurotransmitters

Neurotransmitters can be classified into two broad categories: small-molecule neurotransmitters and neuropeptides. Small-molecule neurotransmitters create rapid synaptic action. Large-molecule neurotransmitters, called "neuropeptides," initiate slow and often ongoing synaptic activity.

For a molecule to be classified as a neurotransmitter it must:
- be present within the presynaptic neuron,
- be released in response to a presynaptic electrical signal that causes calcium to flow into the presynaptic ending (synaptic bouton), and
- activate postsynaptic cell receptors.

Neurons often contain and release different neurotransmitters. A neuron may have small and large molecule neurotransmitters packaged in separate vesicles. These can be released separately or simultaneously. For example, low-level stimulation often releases small-molecule neurotransmitters like glutamate, the primary excitatory neurotransmitter. On the other hand, high-level stimulation will release large molecule neurotransmitters, such as the neuropeptide "substance P," which is involved in the perception of pain.

Two-part synapse

A two-part synapse is defined as having a presynaptic neuron, a postsynaptic neuron, and a synaptic cleft between the neurons.

Chemical synapse communication between the presynaptic neuron and postsynaptic neuron is based on a sequence (Figure 8.10).
- A presynaptic neuron becomes activated sending an electrical current, called an "action potential," down its axon membrane reaching axon endings, called "axon terminals" or "synaptic boutons."

- The action potential causes channels to open in the synaptic bouton through which calcium ions flow into the presynaptic terminal.
- Calcium influx causes vesicles to fuse with the presynaptic membrane.
- Vesicles release neurotransmitter into the space between the neurons called a "synaptic cleft."
- Neurotransmitter diffuses into the synaptic cleft and binds with chemical receptor molecules on the postsynaptic membrane.
- Receptor molecules respond by opening or closing postsynaptic channels causing changes in the excitability of the postsynaptic neuron. (When the postsynaptic neuron reaches a certain level of excitability it will send an action potential along its axon.)
- Neurotransmitter is freed from receptor molecules to be taken up by the neuron, or to be taken up by surrounding glial cells, or to diffuse into the extracellular space.
- Vesicular membrane is retrieved from the presynaptic membrane to be reused by the presynaptic neuron to package more neurotransmitter.

The time it takes for the neurotransmitter to be released, bind to receptors, and have an effect is less than a millionth of a second.

Neurotransmitter receptor channels

There are two kinds of neurotransmitter receptor channels, direct and indirect, referred to respectively as "ionotropic receptors" and "metabotropic receptors."

Ionotropic receptor

A direct channel receptor is also known as an "ionotropic receptor." When a neurotransmitter binds with a direct channel, the channel opens, allowing ions to flow directly through the channel. Direct channels are called "ionotropic receptors" or "ion channels" and are very fast receptors, operating on millisecond time frames.

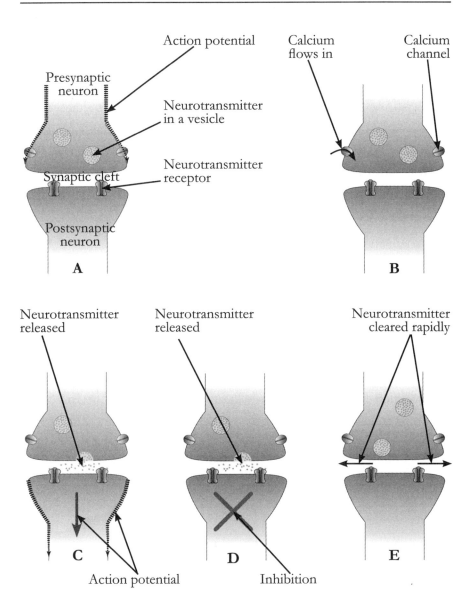

Figure 8.10. Chemical synapse. **A:** Action potential travels down presynaptic membrane. **B:** Calcium channels open allowing calcium to flow into presynaptic neuron. **C:** Neurotransmitter released into the synaptic cleft binds to postsynaptic neuron receptors, and an action potential is sent along membrane, or **D:** inhibition of the postsynaptic neuron occurs. **E:** Neurotransmitter cleared rapidly from the synaptic cleft.

Metabotropic receptor

An "indirect channel" receptor is also known as a "metabotropic receptor." When a neurotransmitter binds with an indirect channel, it causes a chemical (metabolic) change to take place within the receiving neuron. This change can lead to opening or closing of ion channels. Metabotropic receptors are slower than ionotropic receptors, operating within time frames of milliseconds to minutes.

Neuron signaling is constantly modified

Neurons have both types of receptors and are constantly, through receptor reactions, interacting with other neurons, glial cells, and substances within interstitial fluid. This allows neuron signaling to be modified by other cells both locally and at a distance and helps optimize and synchronize neural network signaling.

Electrical synapse

Electrical synapses are formed by areas of direct connection between neurons through which electrical currents flow. An electrical synapse consists of a group of small passageways in cell membranes, called "gap junctions," that directly connect the cytoplasm of two cells. Gap junctions couple together a large group of similar cells to help synchronize their cell activity. Electrical synapses work by ions flowing through gap junctions due to passive diffusion (Figure 8.11). Recent research shows that electrical and molecular flows can take place in both directions between neurons at the electrical synapse.

CHAPTER 8 NEURONS, SYNAPSES, AND ASTROCYTES

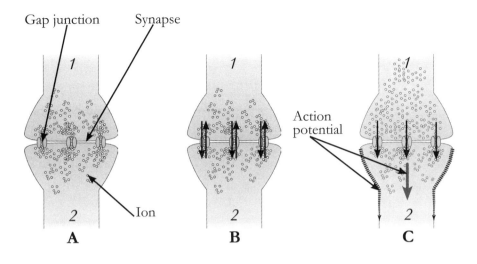

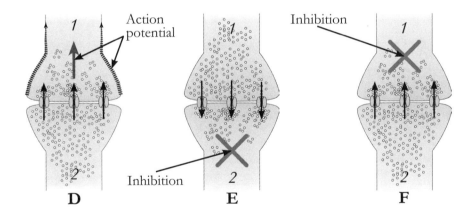

Figure 8.11. Electrical synapse. An ion is an atom or a molecule with either a positive or negative charge. **A:** An electrical synapse. Ions flowing between neurons through gap junctions due to passive diffusion. **B:** Ions have a bidirectional flow (can flow from **1** to **2** or flow from **2** to **1**). **C:** Ions flowing from **1** to **2** are causing an action potential in **2**. **D:** Ions flowing from **2** to **1** are causing an action potential in **1**. **E:** Ions flowing from **1** to **2** are causing inhibition in **2**. **F:** Ions flowing from **2** to **1** are causing inhibition in **1**.

145

Astrocytes and the three-part synapse model

The most abundant non-neuronal cell in the CNS is a glial cell called an "astrocyte." One primary function of astrocytes takes place at the synapse where they help support, modify, enhance, and organize signaling. This has led to the idea of the three-part synapse, also known as the "tripartite synapse."

Three parts of the tripartite synapse are: presynaptic neuron, postsynaptic neuron, and astrocytes encasing the synapse (Figure 8.12). The presynaptic neuron and postsynaptic neuron are covered in the preceding section. The focus of this section is to discuss astrocyte contributions to synaptic function.

Astrocytes influence neural signaling

Astrocytes are involved in neurological signaling in five main ways. These are discussed in the following sections:
- metabolic support,
- gliotransmitters,
- glial neurotransmitter receptors,
- astrocyte calcium waves, and
- potassium spatial buffering.

Metabolic support

Neurons have two main sources of energy: blood glucose and lactate. Glucose enters the CNS interstitium by passing through two barriers. The first barrier is the blood-brain barrier, which has glucose transporters allowing glucose to enter the perivascular space (Figure 8.13). The second barrier is formed by astrocyte end-feet surrounding blood vessels (perivascular glial limiting membrane). These end-feet have glucose transporters through which glucose enters the astrocyte (Figure 8.13). Once the glucose enters the astrocyte, the astrocyte will do one or more of the following:

- transfer glucose through channels locally into the extracellular space to be used by neurons and other glial cells,
- transport glucose to other regions by way of the glial syncytium,
- use glucose for its own energy needs, and
- store glucose as a converted energy substrate (glycogen).

Neurons do not store glycogen, which is the storage form of glucose. On the other hand, astrocytes do store glucose as glycogen. Astrocytes are the largest energy reserve in the brain.

During resting-state neural activity, uptake of glucose by neurons and astrocytes is equal. During periods of neural signaling, glucose is primarily taken up by astrocytes. Astrocytes respond to neural signaling by quickly converting stored glycogen into lactate and then transporting it to neurons as an energy boost (Figure 8.14). Without this astrocyte energy assistance, neurons would quickly run out of energy and lose their ability to signal.

Astrocytes surrounding synapses are involved in providing neurons with glutamine (Figure 8.15), which is used by neurons to produce both glutamate and gamma aminobutyric acid (GABA). In the CNS, glutamate is the primary excitatory neurotransmitter, and GABA is the principle inhibitory neurotransmitter.

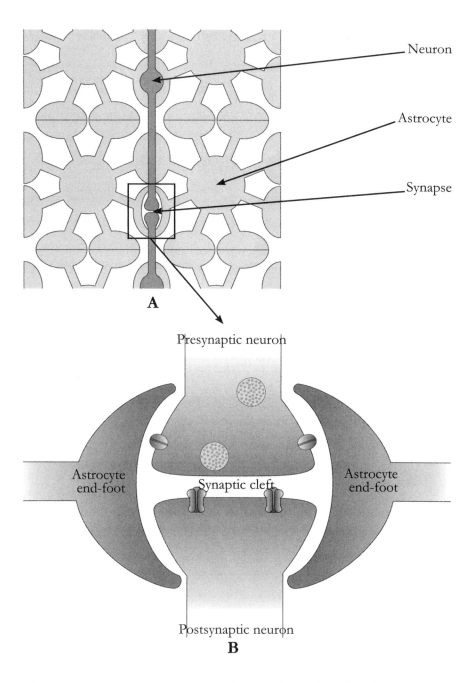

Figure 8.12. Three-part synapse. **A:** An illustration showing astrocytes encasing a synapse. **B:** Detail of a three-part synapse.

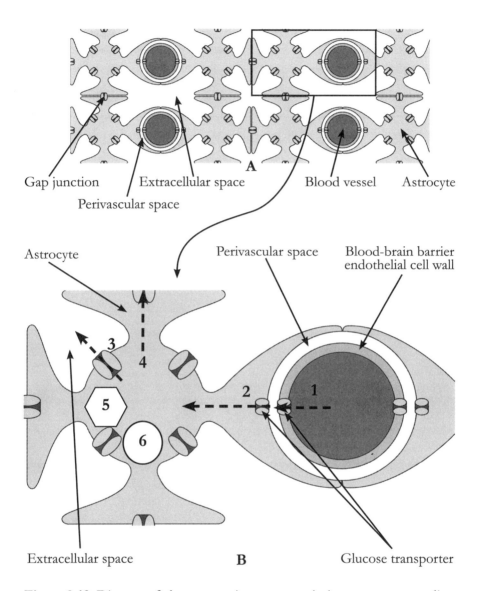

Figure 8.13. Diagram of glucose entering astrocyte. **A:** Astrocytes surrounding blood vessels. **B:** Glucose enters astrocyte. **1:** Glucose is transported through the blood-brain barrier endothelial cell into the perivascular space. **2:** Glucose is transported from the perivascular space into an astrocyte. **3:** Glucose leaves the astrocyte to enter the extracellular space. **4:** Glucose flows through gap junction channels into other astrocytes. **5:** Glucose is used for the astrocyte's energy needs. **6:** Glucose is stored within the astrocyte.

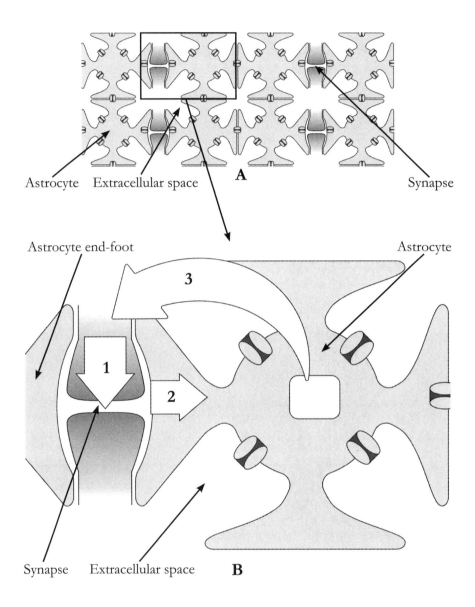

Figure 8.14. Diagram of an astrocyte supplying a neuron with an energy substrate. **A:** Astrocytes surrounding synapses. **B:** Astrocyte sends a neuron energy substrate. **1:** Neuron signals. **2:** Astrocyte senses neural signaling and converts stored glycogen into lactate. **3:** Astrocyte sends lactate to the active neuron.

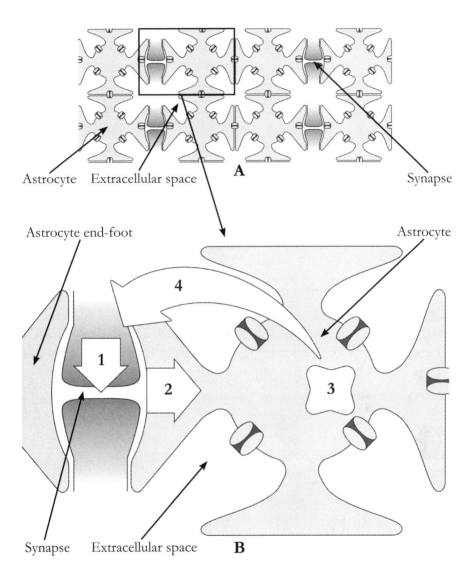

Figure 8.15. Diagram of an astrocyte supplying a neuron with a neurotransmitter substrate. **A:** Astrocytes surrounding synapses. **B:** Glutamate-glutamine shuttle. **1:** Neuron releases glutamate into the synaptic cleft. **2:** Astrocyte absorbs excess glutamate from the synaptic cleft. **3:** Converts glutamate into glutamine and stores it. **4:** Supplies the neuron with glutamine as needed by the neuron. The neuron will then convert glutamine into glutamate. This process is called the "glutamate-glutamine shuttle."

Gliotransmitters

Astrocytes release molecules, called "gliotransmitters," that can bind to both presynaptic and postsynaptic receptors (Figure 8.16). The gliotransmitters modify neural signaling by influencing the excitability of neurons. The major gliotransmitters are: glutamate, GABA, adenosine triphosphate (ATP), and D-serine. Gliotransmitters match the specific neurotransmitters of the synapse they surround.

Glial neurotransmitter receptors

Astrocytes have receptors for a wide range of neurotransmitters. The receptors match the encased neuron's type of neurotransmitter. Glial receptors are activated by neurotransmitters released into a synaptic cleft. Glial receptors then modify glial internal processes creating a response in the astrocytes, which in turn modify neural processes (Figure 8.17).

Astrocyte calcium waves

Each astrocyte forms on average 30,000 gap junctions per cell. Astrocytes make these interconnections primarily with other astrocytes. Astrocytes may also form gap junctions with oligodendrocytes, axons, synapses, blood vessels, the pia mater membrane, the ventricles, and some neurons. This interconnected matrix of glial cells, formed by gap junctions, is referred to as the "glial syncytium."

One primary way astrocytes surrounding synapses respond to synaptic activity is to release internal (intracellular) stores of calcium. This calcium release is a means of communication between glial cells (intracellular communication) and is often referred to as "astrocyte calcium waves" (Figure 8.18).

Glial syncytial communication can synchronize the activity of near and distant neurological networks as well as synchronize glial activity. Syncytial processes are modified by both neural signaling and glial communication. Glia are active partners of neurons, and they have reciprocal supportive roles in all nervous system activity. The glial syncytium can also be viewed as a parallel memory and computing network working in harmony with neural networks. Combined networks of neurons and glial cells vastly expand the capacity of the brain and spinal cord to process and store information.

Potassium spatial buffering

A vital element of optimal neuron signaling is the chemical composition of the extracellular space (ECS) surrounding neurons and glial cells. Potassium is involved in neural signaling. The amount of potassium inside and outside neurons must be constantly and precisely controlled or impaired neural signaling can take place.

For example, large shifts in the neuron's outside-to-inside balance of sodium and potassium takes place when a neuron sends an electrical signal along its axon (action potential). Potassium increases in the ECS during signaling. If too much potassium stays in the ECS then the neuron may signal excessively, chaotically, or not at all. Excess potassium must be constantly removed from the ECS on a moment-to-moment basis. The primary way this takes place is through astrocytes.

Oligodendrocytes encase CNS axons in a fatty insulation called "myelin." CNS myelin is discussed in Chapter 11, "Oligodendrocytes and myelin." Myelin is arranged along the length of an axon in sections. Small gaps, called "nodes of Ranvier," exist between myelin sections (Figure 8.19).

Astrocyte end-feet send microvilli processes, called "perinodal processes," into nodes of Ranvier (Figure 8.19). Perinodal processes have potassium channels through which excess potassium flows into an astrocyte. This potassium will be stored by the astrocyte to then be released back into the nodal space as needed, sent through the glial syncytium to either an area of low potassium concentration, or sent to the venous system to exit the CNS (Figure 8.20). This flow of excess potassium into, out of, or through astrocytes is called "potassium spatial buffering."

Optimizing CNS function

Astrocytes have receptors for almost all neurotransmitters and neurohormones that are involved in nervous system signaling. Astrocytes are constantly sensing and responding to synaptic and neural network activity, and they modulate synaptic and neural network signaling by releasing gliotransmitters that match the neurons they surround. Astrocytes also take up neurotransmitters from the synaptic cleft so that excessive amounts of neurotransmitter do not accumulate in the synapse, which could lead to chaotic signaling or even neuronal death due to hyperexcitability. CNS function results from an interrelated, interdependent, and coordinated millisecond to millisecond collaboration between neurons, glial cells, and the substances within the ECS.

Neurons nestle in a structural matrix of astrocytes. Neural dysfunction can occur when this astrocyte matrix is distorted because form and function are interrelated and interdependent. I will discuss how deformation of astrocyte channels can alter neural signaling as an example of how form distortion leads to dysfunction.

Astrocyte uptake of neurotransmitter is one significant way the control of synaptic neurotransmitter and neural signaling takes place. Proteins of a particular form create astrocyte channels through which pass excess synaptic neurotransmitter (ESN). ESN travels from the synapse, through astrocyte channels, and then into astrocyte end-feet (Figure 8.14).

The flow of ESN may be obstructed when astrocyte channels are deformed, causing harmful neurotransmitter buildup within the synaptic cleft. This buildup can cause neurons to signal when they should be resting, causing unregulated, or chaotic signaling. Or ESN can cause excessive or uncontrolled inhibition that makes it abnormally difficult for neurons to signal. Uncontrolled inhibition can cause chaotic signaling or a shut down of signaling.

Disturbed signaling can lead to many conditions, some of which are: seizure, memory impairment, anxiety, hyperactivity, dizziness, tinnitus, developmental delays, or motor impairment.

Astrocyte stressors occur in response to a range of problems, such as infection, toxicity, blood flow alterations, or biomechanical strain. Astrocyte adverse biomechanical stress can occur in response to stressful patterns generated by the CNS parenchyma or harmful patterns transmitted into the parenchyma through the pia-glial interface (Chapter 4, "Pia-glial interface").

Craniosacral therapy techniques can lessen astrocyte stress by transmitting corrective forces through the pia-glial interface. These corrective forces can help improve astrocyte form, and this can lead to enhanced astrocyte function. Improved astrocyte shape and function contributes to enhancing the work of neurons, astrocytes, and other glial cells, which can lead to improved CNS health and function.

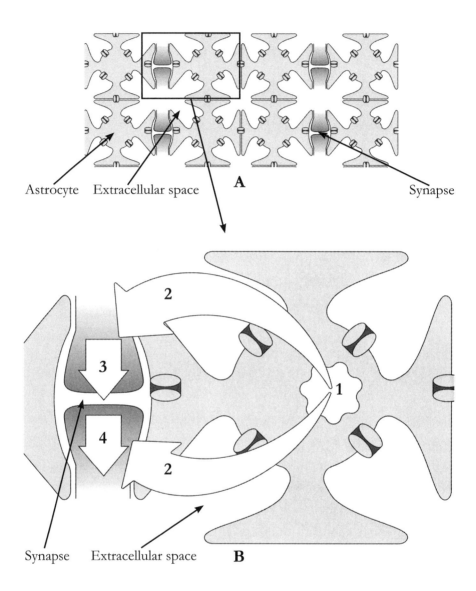

Figure 8.16. Diagram of astrocyte release of gliotransmitters. **A:** Astrocytes surrounding synapses. **B:** Release of gliotransmitters. **1:** Astrocyte storage of gliotransmitter. **2:** Astrocyte release of gliotransmitter. Neural response to the released gliotransmitter follows. **3:** Initiate the release of neurotransmitter into the synaptic cleft by a presynaptic neuron. **4:** Initiate an action potential in a postsynaptic neuron.

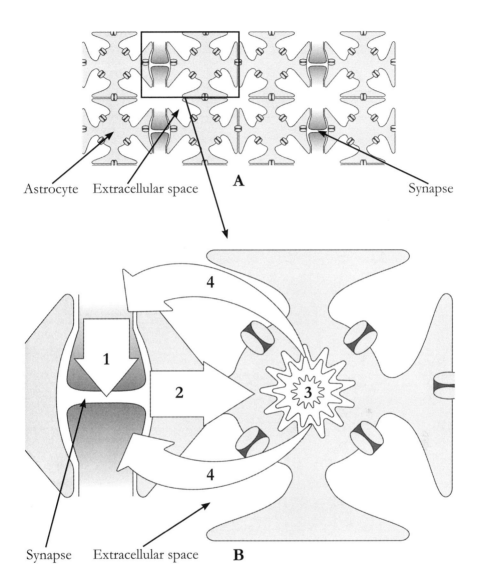

Figure 8.17. Diagram of an astrocyte stimulated by neurotransmitter. **A:** Astrocytes surrounding synapses. **B:** Astrocyte response to neurotransmitter. **1:** Neurotransmitter is released into the synaptic cleft. **2:** Glial neurotransmitter receptor is activated. **3:** Astrocyte internal processes are modified by the neurotransmitter receptor stimulation. **4:** Astrocyte may respond by releasing substances that modify neural processes of either the presynaptic or postsynaptic neuron.

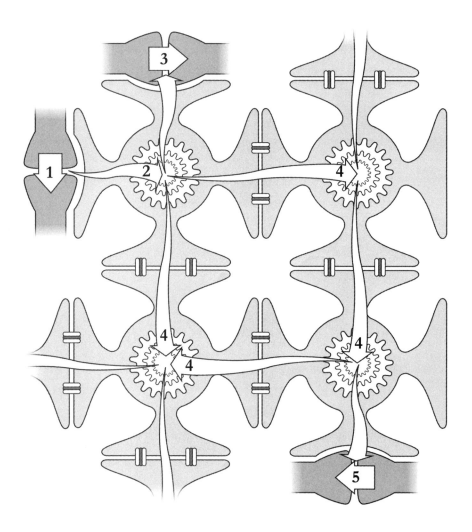

Figure 8.18. Astrocyte calcium waves in response to synaptic signaling. **1:** Neural signaling. **2:** Astrocyte senses neural activity, which causes a release of intracellular calcium. **3:** Calcium can stimulate neural processes in the astrocyte's local domain. **4:** Waves of calcium flow in between astrocytes. **5:** Calcium waves may modify distant neural processes.

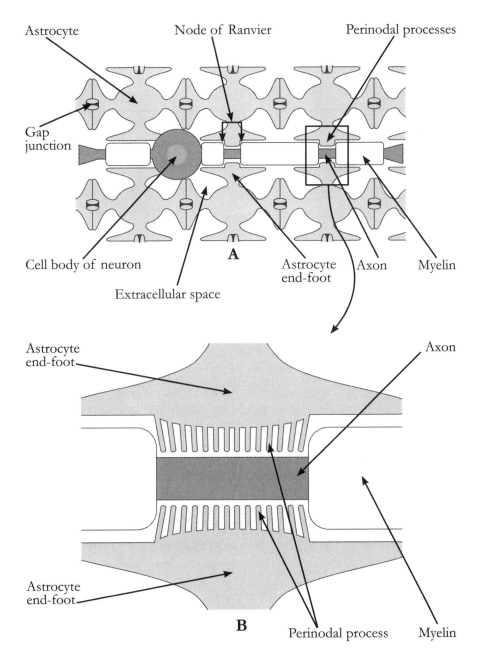

Figure 8.19. Astrocyte perinodal processes. **A:** Astrocytes surrounding a neuron and myelin sheath. **B:** Detail of perinodal processes extending into a node of Ranvier.

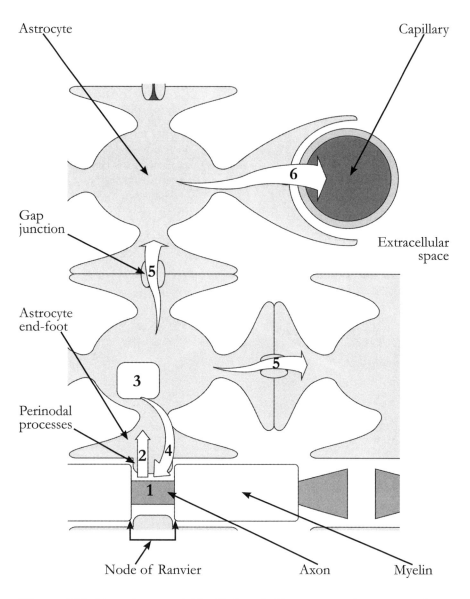

Figure 8.20. Potassium spatial buffering. **1:** Excess potassium accumulates within the node of Ranvier. **2:** Potassium flows through perinodal processes into an astrocyte. **3:** Astrocyte stores potassium. **4:** Potassium released into node of Ranvier as needed. **5:** Astrocyte transports potassium to other astrocytes through gap junctions. **6:** Potassium transported from the astrocyte into a blood vessel at the capillary level.

Chapter 9

The extracellular space and transmission types

*H*ow does the central nervous system (CNS) receive, use, and store information? Are neurons the only cells involved in CNS information processing?

Neurons, glial cells, and substances within the extracellular space take part in transmitting and storing information. The size, shape, and composition of the extracellular space is involved directly in two forms of information transmission. In this chapter we will first discuss the extracellular space and then CNS transmission types.

The extracellular space

The total volume of the CNS is comprised of:
- cells and blood vessels (80 percent of the total volume), and
- extracellular space (20 percent).

There are tiny gaps between the neurons and glial cells in the CNS. Together those minute spaces form a convoluted and complex system of small, interconnected tube-like passageways that span the entire CNS interstitium. This labyrinthine network of channels is called the extracellular space (ECS) (Figure 9.1 and Figure 9.2).

The ECS is crowded with:
- interstitial fluid,
- ions,
- neurotransmitters,
- metabolites,
- peptides,
- neurohormones,
- neuroactive substances,
- gliotransmitters,
- gliomodulators, and
- molecules of the extracellular matrix (ECM).

Molecules keep the ECS open

ECM molecules, especially glycosaminoglycans, maintain the open shape of the ECS in two ways:
- glycosaminoglycans are arranged in such a way that they repel each other, keeping the ECS from collapsing in upon itself; and
- glycosaminoglycans draw water into the ECS, further expanding its minute channels.

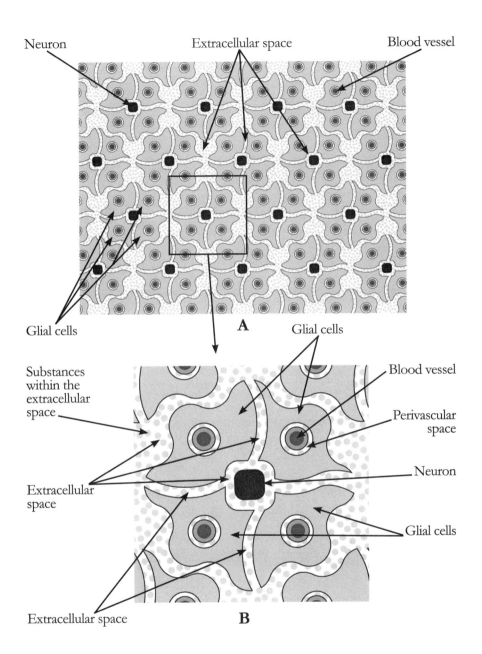

Figure 9.1. The extracellular space. **A:** Diagram of the extracellular space, glia, neurons, and blood vessels. **B:** Detail of the extracellular space.

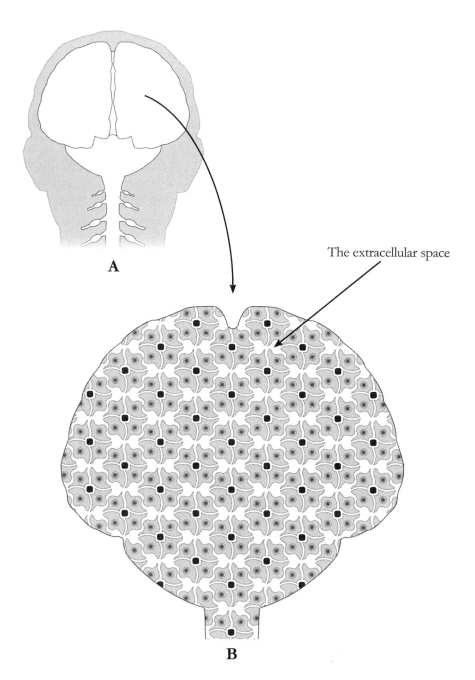

Figure 9.2. The extracellular space. **A:** Anterior view of the brain and a portion of the spinal cord. **B:** The extracellular space.

CNS passageways

Substances must be able to enter, flow through, and exit the CNS interstitium. The ECS tubules provide the sole passageway for this essential movement. Cerebrospinal fluid, water, nutrients, glucose, oxygen, and other substances need to enter and flow throughout the ECS to support the metabolic needs of neurons and glia. Substances such as inflammatory molecules, excess ions, waste products, and toxins need to flow through the ECS in order to exit and be removed from the CNS.

Glia constantly alter ECS shape

Key to the health of the CNS is the maintenance of open ECS passageways. Glial cells are constantly changing form while fulfilling their normal activities (Figure 9.3). As an example, when neurotransmitter is released into a synaptic cleft, astrocyte end-feet absorb water from the cleft. This helps to tighten the astrocyte end-feet encapsulation of the synapse to assure excess neurotransmitter does not escape into the surrounding ECS. As astrocytes take in water, they swell slightly. This water either flows back into the synaptic cleft, flows through gap junctions to adjacent astrocytes, flows into the ECS, or is reabsorbed into the venous system. As astrocytes transport water to other astrocytes, or release water, they shrink slightly. This is one example of a multitude of glial processes during which glial size is always increasing and decreasing.

Pathological processes may also cause glia to either shrink or swell. Ongoing swelling is harmful because it places excessive pressure upon neurons and glia and reduces the size of the ECS. When the passageways of the ECS diminish in size, obstructions occur.

Substances begin to accumulate causing excessive cell stress and chaotic signaling. Nutrients and neuroactive substances then cannot reach their target destinations.

Everything each cell in the CNS needs in order to survive and function must pass within the ECS. If the ECS shrinks in size, becomes clogged with debris or is inflamed, then the consequences can be drastic.

Craniosacral therapy techniques can help normalize the shape of the ECS by transmitting corrective forces through the pia-glial interface (Figure 4.21 and Figure 4.22). Unobstructed ECS aids the flow of ECS substances and interstitial fluid that are essential to almost all CNS processes, including CNS communication.

Transmission types

There are four ways in which CNS cells communicate, they are:
- wired transmission,
- extracellular volume transmission,
- ephaptic coupling, and
- intracellular volume transmission.

Together these four means of transmission create an extraordinarily efficient, integrated, flexible, dynamic, and broad signaling system for the CNS. The CNS can then effectively respond to, control, organize, and store information received via those signals, and thus manage mind and body functions.

Wired transmission

Wired transmission is a form of nervous system communication that takes place when one cell communicates with another cell, which is also known as "one-to-one signaling" (Figure 9.4 and Figure 9.5). Wired transmission is the form of signaling described in the Neuron Doctrine. It is an extremely fast signal transmission between neurons and lasts from milliseconds to a few seconds.

CHAPTER 9   THE EXTRACELLULAR SPACE AND TRANSMISSION TYPES

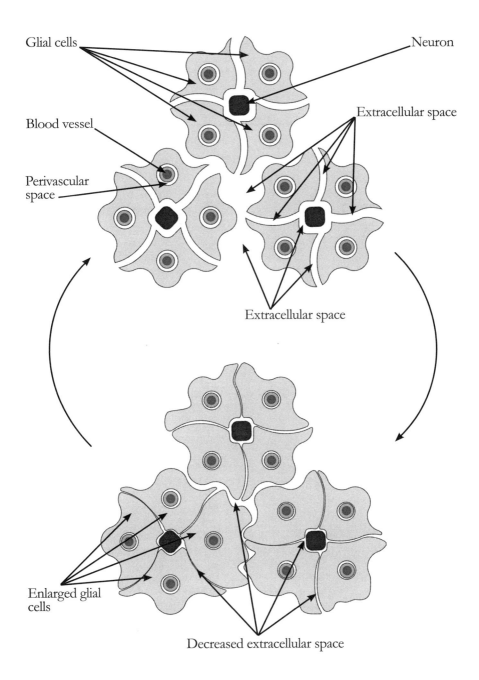

Figure 9.3. Glial cells are constantly changing shape, which changes the shape of the extracellular space.

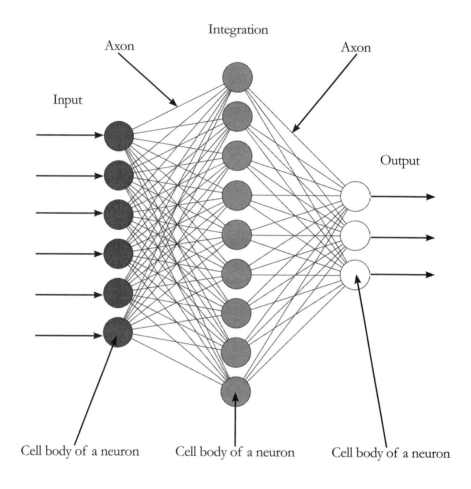

Figure 9.4. A diagram of a neural network.

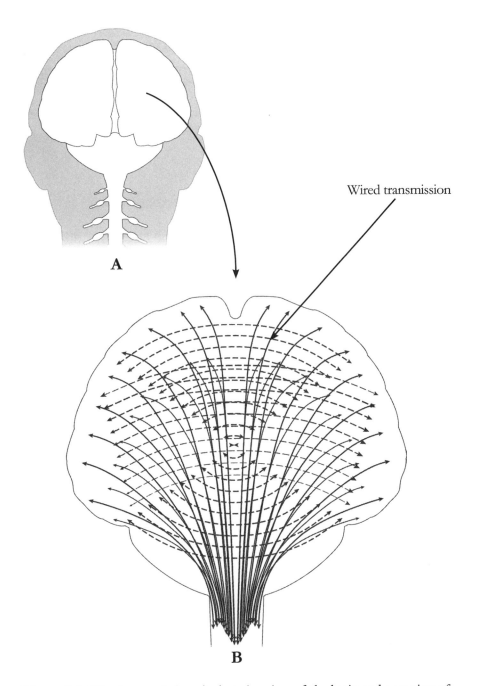

Figure 9.5. Wired transmission. **A:** Anterior view of the brain and a portion of the spinal cord. **B:** Diagram of wired transmission.

Extracellular volume transmission

Extracellular volume transmission (EVT) is slower than wired transmission and can have effects lasting for minutes, hours, or days. Some research suggests effects can last for years.

EVT occurs when signaling substances that are outside of cells spread (diffuse) by flowing within the extracellular space. This is called "one-to-many" communication because one cell affects many other cells (Figure 9.6 and Figure 9.7).

"Neuroactive" substances flow throughout the ECS either directly or indirectly affecting the way neurons and glia function. Both neurons and glia release neuroactive substances into the ECS that diffuse locally and distant from the release sites.

EVT occurs between neurons or between neurons and glial cells. It is an extremely important means of synchronizing local and distant neuroglial networks.

The size and shape of the ECS determines the movement of its substances. Adverse modification of the ECS could alter normal volume transmission because the neurotransmitters, neuromodulators, gliotransmitters, or gliomodulators may not be able to reach their intended targets. This could impair neuron signaling and glial function, which could lead to functional deficits and neuron/glial damage.

Molecules produced by both neurons and glia have been shown to create functional groups of neurons, glia, and axon tracts by creating avenues within the ECS that direct the flow of substances towards, as well as away from, specific areas.

Ephaptic coupling

Local electrical fields are produced when neurons signal and glial cells communicate. These fields affect surrounding cells and are a form of extracellular volume transmission. Neural and glial electrical fields spread to other neurons and glia in such a way that they synchronize or modify neuroglial activity. It is another form of "one-to-many" communication (Figure 9.8 and Figure 9.9).

Intracellular volume transmission

When diffusion or flow of signaling substances, typically calcium (often referred to as "calcium waves"), occurs inside and between astrocytes, it is called "intracellular volume transmission." It takes place primarily through gap junctions interconnecting the glial syncytium. It is another form of "one-to-many" communication (Figure 9.10 and Figure 9.11).

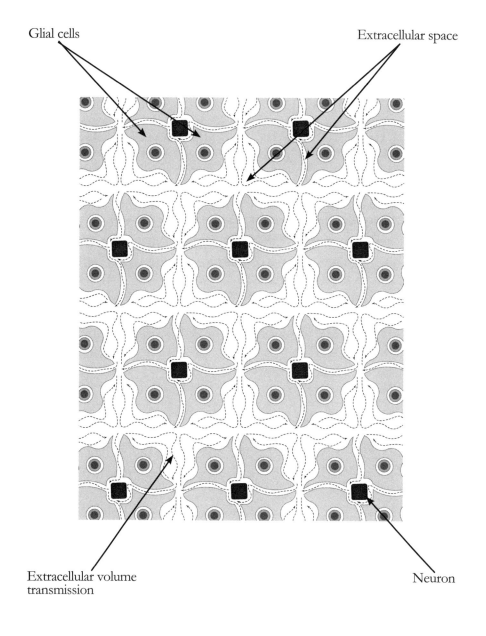

Figure 9.6. Diagram of extracellular volume transmission.

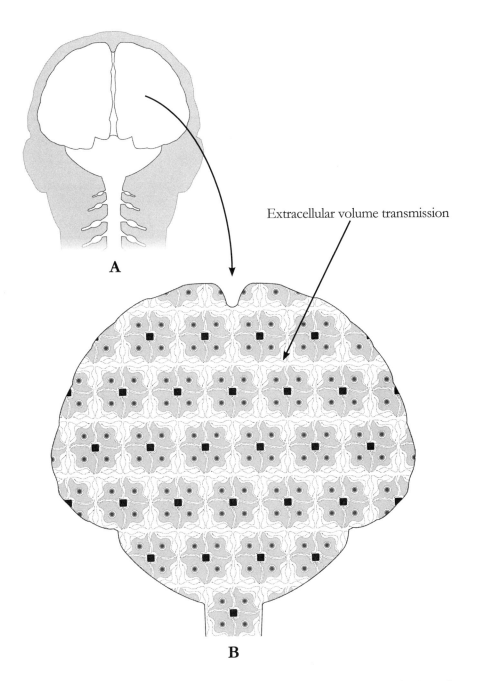

Figure 9.7. Extracellular volume transmission. **A:** Anterior view of the brain and a portion of the spinal cord. **B:** Extracellular volume transmission.

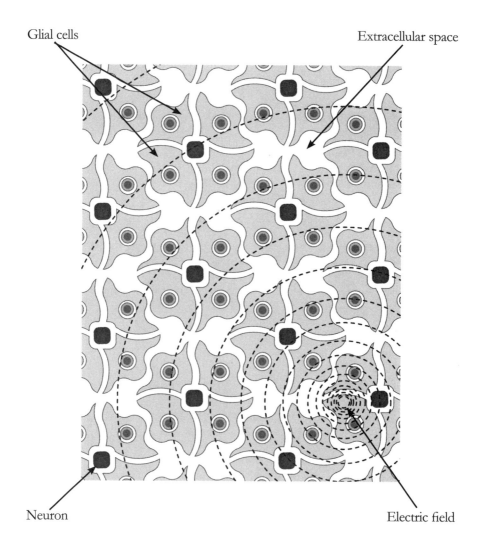

Figure 9.8. Diagram of ephaptic coupling.

CHAPTER 9 THE EXTRACELLULAR SPACE AND TRANSMISSION TYPES

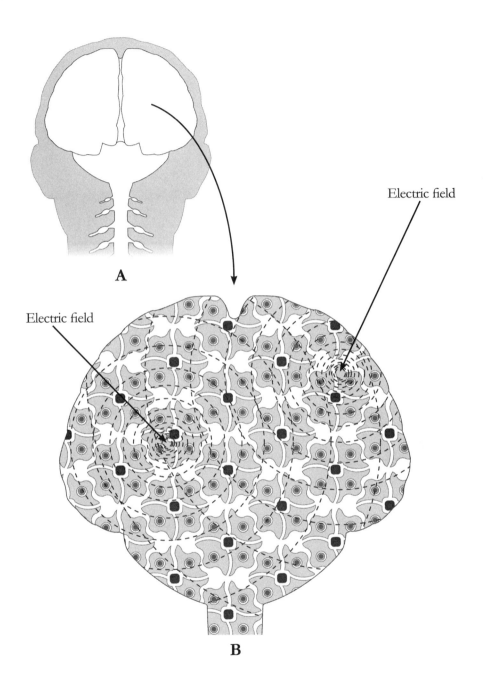

Figure 9.9. Ephaptic coupling. **A:** Anterior view of the brain and a portion of the spinal cord. **B:** Ephaptic coupling electric fields.

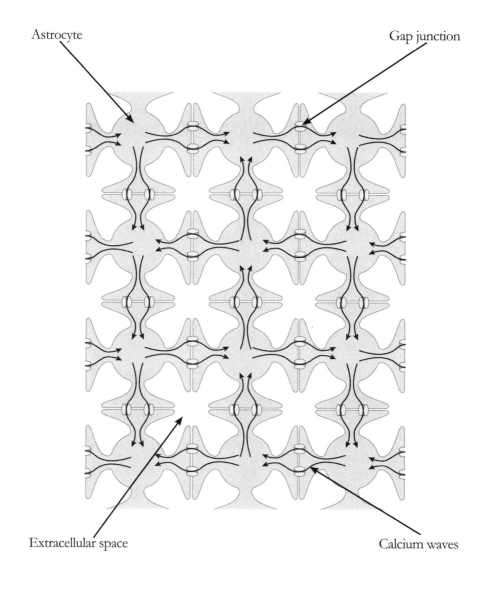

Figure 9.10. Diagram of intracellular volume transmission.

CHAPTER 9   THE EXTRACELLULAR SPACE AND TRANSMISSION TYPES

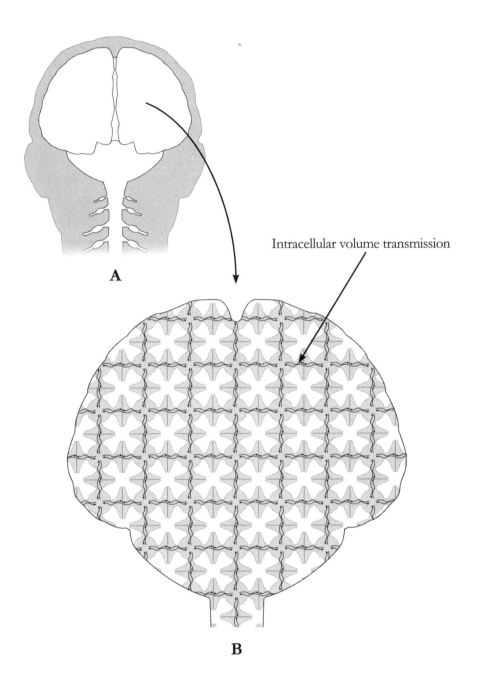

Figure 9.11. Intracellular volume transmission. **A:** Anterior view of the brain and a portion of the spinal cord. **B:** Intracellular volume transmission.

Chapter 10

The blood-brain barrier and the neurovascular unit

The central nervous system (CNS) is the most sensitive and highly-regulated tissue within the body. The composition and timing of substances entering the interstitium from blood must be precisely controlled in order to maintain optimal homeostasis.

The "blood-brain barrier" regulates the types of substances allowed entry into the CNS. The "neurovascular unit" links the flow of blood substances passing into the interstitium with the work of neurons. For example, increased neural signaling requires increased blood flow, decreased neural signaling causes decreased blood flow.

This chapter focuses on the blood-brain barrier, neruovascular unit, and astrocytes that are essential components of both.

The blood-brain barrier

The main function of the blood-brain barrier (BBB) is to guarantee that only certain elements enter the CNS parenchyma from the body's general circulation. This typically assures that the CNS environment can maintain optimal biochemical balance. Blood flow entering the CNS is regulated by the BBB. The BBB exists throughout the entire CNS vascular parenchymal network except at the circumventricular organs.

Blood vessels enter parenchyma

Before discussing the specific components of the BBB, let us look at how blood vessels enter the CNS parenchyma. Blood supply to the brain comes from the internal carotid arteries and the vertebral arteries. Blood supply to the spinal cord comes from the anterior spinal artery, posterior spinal artery, and spinal branches of the segmental arteries. These arteries eventually give rise to smaller arteries that travel within the subarachnoid space. The arteries within the subarachnoid space send branches (arterioles) into the parenchyma through openings within the pia mater membrane. These openings are called "Virchow-Robin spaces" (Figure 10.1).

As an arteriole enters the CNS parenchyma, it is surrounded by both the outer glial limiting membrane astrocyte end-feet and the pia mater membrane (Figure 10.2). The pia mater membrane will end shortly after the blood vessel passes through its Virchow-Robin space, yet the astrocyte end-feet will continue to encase the blood vessel at all levels. The astrocyte end-feet surrounding blood vessels form the perivascular glial limiting membrane, perivascular channels, and part of the BBB.

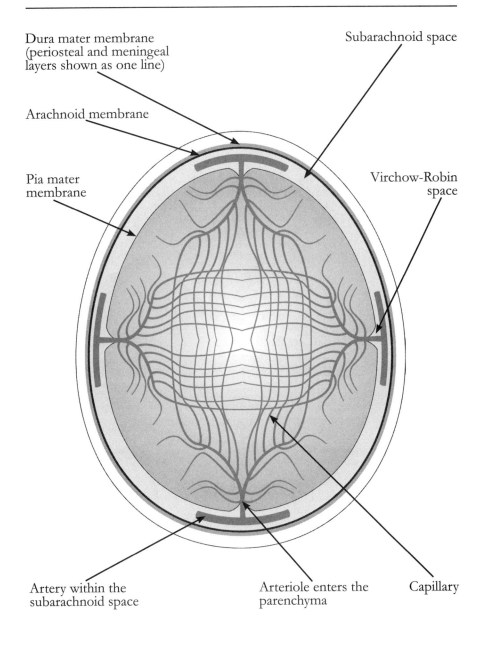

Figure 10.1. Transverse section of the brain showing arteries within the subarachnoid space and arterioles entering the brain parenchyma by traveling through Virchow-robin spaces.

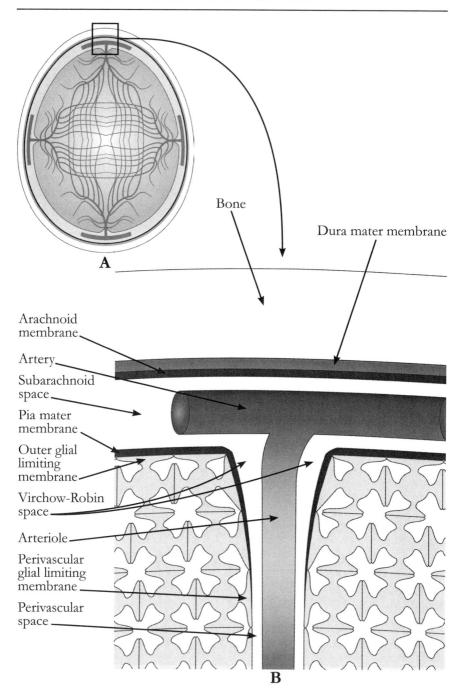

Figure 10.2. A: Transverse brain section. **B:** Detail of an arteriole entering the brain parenchyma through the Virchow-Robin space.

BBB components

BBB is comprised of (Figure 10.3 and Figure 10.4):
- endothelial cells,
- basement membrane,
- pericytes, and
- astrocyte end-feet.

Endothelial cells

Capillary vessels within the CNS, where the BBB is found, are comprised of endothelial cells, basement membrane (BM), and pericytes. The inner lining of CNS blood vessels, called "endothelial cells," are different from non-CNS blood vessels primarily in two ways:
- the space in between endothelial cells is much smaller between CNS blood vessels than in non-CNS blood vessels (these small spaces are called "tight junctions"), and
- endothelial cells are much less permeable in CNS blood vessels than non-CNS blood vessels.

Everything entering the CNS from the blood must pass between, or be transported through, BBB endothelial cells. If blood substances are not the correct size, or do not have a specific transporter to carry them through the endothelial cells, then those substances cannot typically enter the CNS.

Basement Membrane

The basement membrane (BM) is a thin sheet of extracellular matrix adhered to the outer surface of endothelial cells. It also lines cavities, organs, and glands throughout the body. Blood vessels reach every speck of the entire body and CNS, and each vessel is encased in BM. BM is classified as fascia and is part of the overall fascial matrix.

CNS BM is a specialized form of extracellular matrix comprised primarily of collagen IV, laminin, perlecan, and nidogen. The BM encases the outer surface of both endothelial cells and pericytes and participates in:
- regulating blood vessel development,
- healing blood vessels,
- forming and maintaining the BBB,
- supporting endothelial cells as a structural matrix,
- regulating the flow of substances through the BBB, and
- providing a CSF efflux pathway.

The BM is a fascial continuum extending from the skin to the depths of the CNS. It is an avenue through which fascial patterns can be transferred deeply into CNS, even all the way to the delicate capillary level. If fascial distortions harm blood vessels, BM, or the BBB, then atypical alterations in CNS blood flow can arise. This may lead to a host of CNS problems because CNS function depends upon continuous and precisely regulated blood flow.

The fascial matrix is not only a continuum through which stressful patterns broadcast. Corrective forces, such as those applied during craniosacral therapy, can be conveyed by a practitioner's hands to the BM. These forces can help restructure blood vessels, and this in turn can help improve blood flow, even in the deepest regions of the brain or spinal cord.

Pericytes

Pericytes are cells that surround the outside of endothelial cells. Pericytes have the ability to contract and release. Channels extend through the basement membrane interlocking pericytes with endothelial cells. This interlock transfers mechanical force from pericyte to endothelium, which alters the diameter of the blood vessel with which it interconnects.

The pericyte channels are also openings through which small molecules travel between pericytes and the endothelial cells they surround. This exchange is a means of communication and activity modification between endothelial cells and pericytes.

Pericytes contribute to:
- vascular development by guiding sprouting vessels,
- modification of vessel wall diameter,
- stabilization of blood vessels,
- survival of endothelial cells,
- communication with other pericytes by integrating vascular physiology and repair processes, and
- macrophage-like (immune cell) activity by engulfing and processing cellular debris and pathogens.

Pericytes also actively interact with all parts of the BBB in modulating blood flow.

BBB astrocytes

Astrocyte end-feet wrap around all CNS capillaries. Therefore, substances moving through capillaries must also move through spaces in between end-feet, or primarily through channels within end-feet, in order to gain entry into the CNS interstitium.

Astrocytes affect the permeability of the BBB by releasing regulatory substances that modify endothelial cells. Endothelial cells modify astrocytes by signaling to them. This signaling regulates receptors and channels within the astrocyte membrane. Instant communication and reciprocal influence between astrocytes, pericytes, and endothelial cells regulate the flow of substances from the blood into the CNS interstitium.

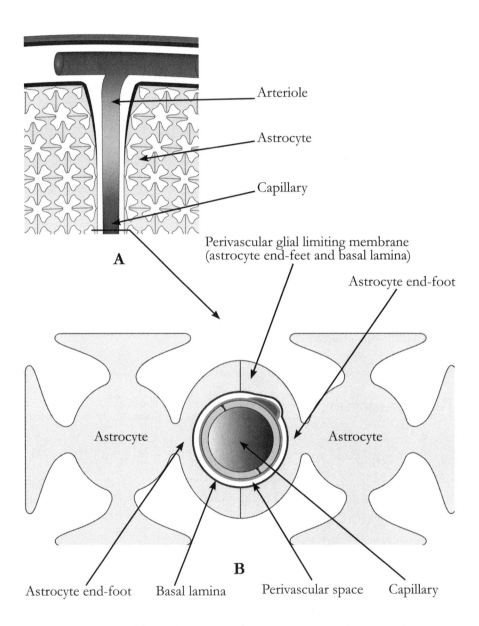

Figure 10.3. Blood-brain barrier. **A:** Arteriole entering the parenchyma. **B:** Cross section of the blood-brain barrier at the micro-vessel level (capillary level).

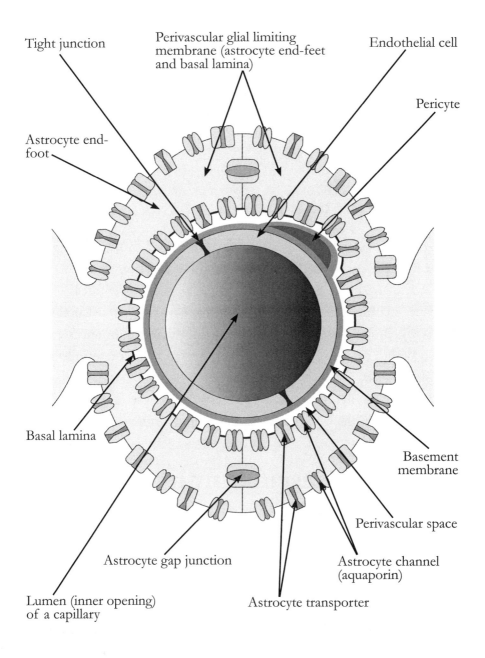

Figure 10.4. Detail of the blood-brain barrier (cross section).

BBB repair

Many CNS insults, such as trauma, stroke, inflammation, or neurodegeneration cause leakiness of the BBB. Often if the harmful insult resolves, then the BBB repairs itself. Astrocytes are essential for BBB repair by producing and secreting a repair molecule called "S-nitrosoglutathione."

Areas without a BBB

Circumventricular organs (CVOs) do not have a BBB, but they do have a BBB encapsulation that forms a separation between each CVO and the brain interstitium. The CVOs are seven areas, called "organs," within the brain that do not have a complete BBB (Figure 10.5). Neurons in these areas can directly detect substances in the blood without needing specific transporters to move these substances across the BBB.

Specialized glial cells, called "tanycytes," cover the CVOs forming a barrier between the CVOs and the brain interstitium.

The neurovascular unit

The structure and function of the CNS depends upon the moment-by-moment controlled flow of substances from the blood into the CNS interstitium. This flow takes place at the capillary level, called the "micro-vessel" level.

Even at rest, CNS cells, primarily neurons, require a huge amount of oxygen, glucose for energy production, and nutrient flow that is supplied by the blood. For instance, the brain comprises 2 percent of the body weight yet requires 20 percent of blood flow, even while at rest, to meet its metabolic needs. It is estimated there are 400 miles of blood vessels in the brain in order to supply microareas with blood flow quickly and efficiently. During wakefulness the amount of energy generated by the brain could power a 24-watt light bulb (Figure 10.6).

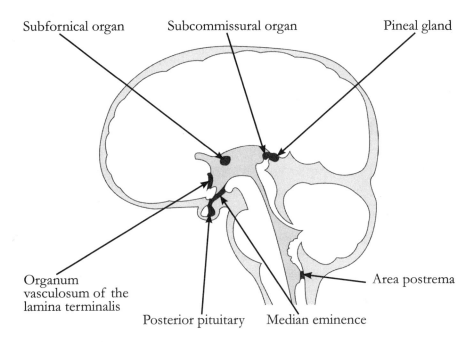

Figure 10.5. Midsagittal section of the brain showing the circumventricular organs.

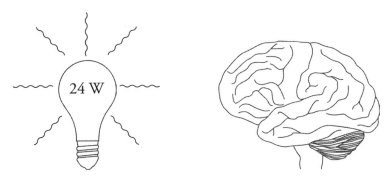

Figure 10.6. The brain can generate enough energy to power a 24-watt light bulb.

Blood flow regulation

CNS blood flow must be precisely regulated in response to activity of cells within very small areas, called "microregions," and throughout the CNS as a whole. This is accomplished through the neurovascular unit (Figure 10.7), which is the interaction of neurons, astrocytes, and BBB cells.

Astrocyte as a functional link

Astrocyte end-feet wrap around synapses and wrap around the entire vasculature of the brain parenchyma, including the BBB. Neurons are linked to their local BBB by way of astrocyte interconnections.

Astrocytes respond to neural activity by instantly communicating this activity to BBB pericytes and endothelial cells in the area of the neuron. This communication regulates the flow of substances from the BBB capillary into the interstitium in three ways:
- stimulating a change in blood vessel diameter, which increases or decreases blood flow,
- modifying active transport of substances through the capillary wall; and
- increasing or decreasing the amount of substances passing through the BBB.

When neuron activity increases, blood flow increases to meet energy, metabolic, and nutrient needs. The volume of substances entering the interstitium from the blood also increase. When neuron activity lessens, local blood flow and substances entering the interstitium decrease in response. There is always a controlled level of both local blood flow and substances entering or leaving the interstitium (Figure 10.8).

Astrocytes are the control cell of the neurovascular unit because they couple synapses with local capillaries (Figure 10.8 and Figure 10.9).

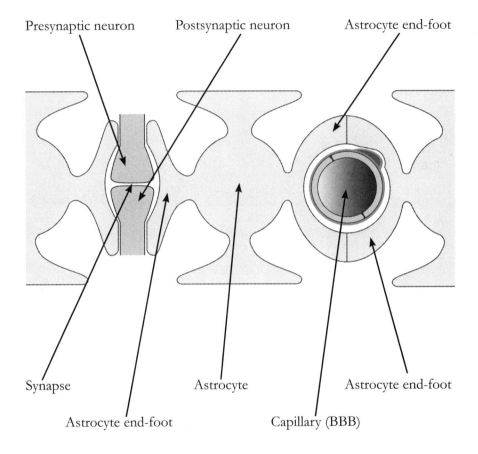

Figure 10.7. The neurovascular unit.

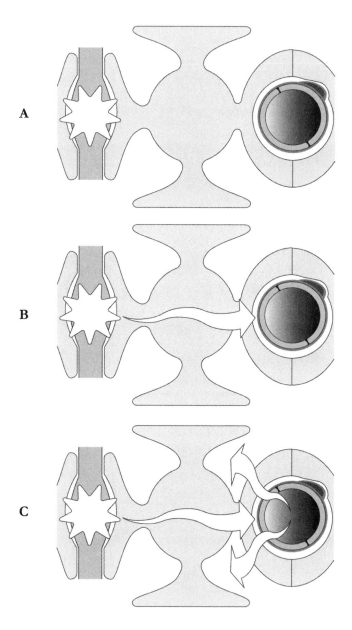

Figure 10.8. Regulation of interstitial blood flow by the neurovascular unit. **A:** Neurotransmitter released into the synaptic cleft. **B:** Astrocyte responds by communicating with the blood-brain barrier capillary. **C:** Blood flow into the interstitium is modified by the capillary components of the blood-brain barrier and the astrocyte.

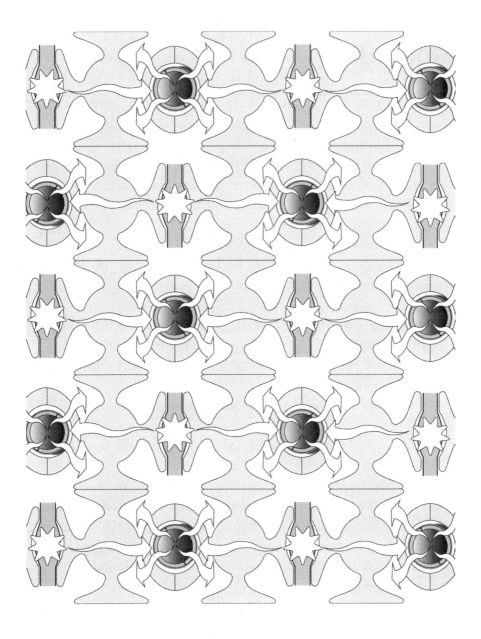

Figure 10.9. Neurovascular units regulating blood flow.

Craniosacral therapy aids CNS blood flow

Fascial strain can distort the meningeal system and the subarachnoid space. A number of blood flow problems can occur in response, such as in the following sequence:
- blood vessels within the subarachnoid space twist, pull, or compress;
- Virchow-Robin spaces tighten, congest, or squeeze arterioles;
- blood vessels transmit strain along epithelial basement membrane to the capillary level;
- capillaries twist, pull, tighten, or excessively open;
- barrier function of the BBB decreases and toxic or infectious substances flow into the interstitium;
- toxicity or infection of the interstitium develops;
- perivascular glial limiting membrane twists, tightens, or excessively opens because blood vessel stress distorts the perivascular space;
- stress in the perivascular glial limiting membrane transfers to the neurovascular unit;
- neurovascular unit becomes dysfunctional;
- blood flow regulation breaks down; and
- neurons, astrocytes, and other glial cells become dysfunctional because metabolic needs are not met.

Some of the problems that may arise due to BBB or neurovascular unit disturbance are: multiple sclerosis, viral or bacterial infection, exhaustion, inflammation, buildup of debris, interstitial congestion, cognitive decline, motor impairment, or post-concussion syndrome.

Craniosacral therapy techniques can lessen meningeal stress and transmit corrective forces through the pia-glial interface. This helps correct the form of blood vessels, the BBB, the perivascular glial limiting membrane, and the neurovascular units. Form correction contributes to decreasing cell stress: structures involved in blood flow or blood flow regulation can heal and normalize their function, improving blood flow and the vitality of the CNS as a whole.

Chapter 11

Oligodendrocytes and myelin

*O*ligodendrocytes are glial cells within the central nervous system (CNS) that produce and maintain insulation (myelin) around neuronal axons.

There are two basic ways to increase the speed and coordination of signals passing through an axon: increase the size of the axon, which is found in invertebrates like the giant squid, or insulate the axon, such as in the vertebrate human nervous system. The fatty insulation around axons, called "myelin," enables the vertebrate nervous system to:

- increase signaling speed;
- enhance timing, coordination, precision, and integration of nerve signals;
- miniaturize the circuitry of nerves and neural networks;

- centralize neurological circuitry into the brain and spinal cord; and
- conserve energy.

One oligodendrocyte can myelinate many axons (Figure 11.1 and Figure 11.2). For instance, a single oligodendrocyte may myelinate sections of 50-60 different axons. As a consequence, damage to one oligodendrocyte will often result in many sites of injury. Myelin has a whitish color because of its lipid content and is often referred to as "white matter." White matter is a combination of myelin and axons. Within the CNS it is known as "substantia alba" and comprises 60 percent of the CNS tissue.

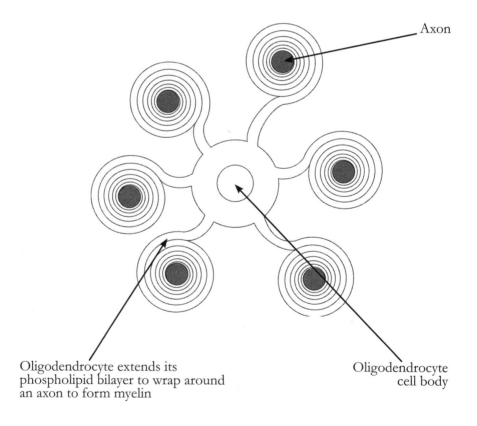

Figure 11.1. One oligodendrocyte myelinating axons (cross section).

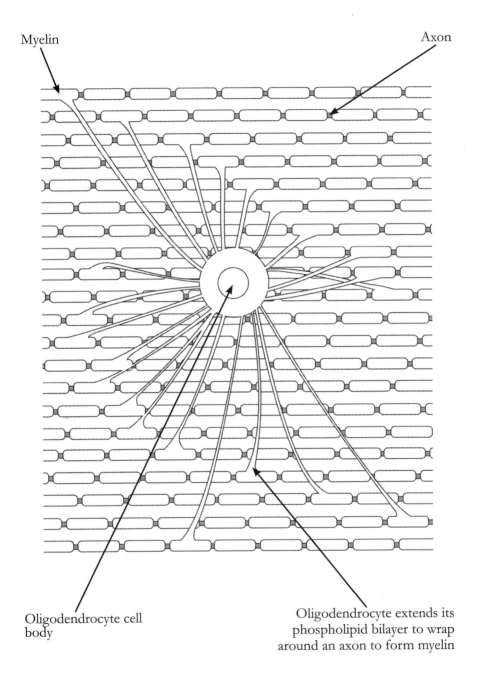

Figure 11.2. Diagram of one oligodendrocyte myelinating many axons.

The process of myelination is influenced by the activity of axons, which is dependent upon neural signaling. Typically myelination begins once an axon reaches its target, forms synapses, and sends electrical signals along its axon. Bundles of axons called "tracts" belong to networks that typically become myelinated at the same time.

Myelination begins when:
- axon activity stimulates secretion of adhesion molecules upon the axon surface so myelin can stick to the axon, which is essential in order for myelin to wrap around the axon;
- signaling molecules, such as glutamate and adenosine triphosphate (ATP), are released from active axons, which begin and then regulate the myelination process; and
- ATP that is released by active axons stimulates astrocytes to release molecules that promote myelination.

Myelination in the CNS is also regulated by molecules within the extracellular space (ECS), such as myelin growth factors. Oligodendrocytes are in direct contact with the ECS. In this way myelination is coordinated through extracellular volume transmission, which synchronizes local and broad network myelination.

Axons are myelinated when they reach a certain size. Oligodendrocytes recognize when an axon reaches a specific diameter, called the "critical diameter." Myelination occurs only when axons reach this critical diameter.

The speed and synchrony of communication within and between neurological networks is critical in all aspects of function, such as learning, movement, and creative thought. One of the most important structures affecting speed and coordination of neuron signaling is myelin.

Speed of signaling is not the only part of nerve conduction that is critical. Timing of signals reaching synapses is also of utmost importance in the sequencing of neuron signaling because changes in synaptic activity last only milliseconds. Myelin forms itself so that simultaneous impulses from multiple points of varying distances can reach the same place at the same time.

The body is always trying to work at optimal function with the least expenditure of energy. Myelin allows neurological signaling to take place with the least amount of energy because it stops energy leakage out of the neuron, and it is constructed in such a way that electrical conduction takes place by jumping between nodes of Ranvier (Figure 11.3).

Myelin is the body substance that allowed the vertebrate nervous system to grow into a complex, intricate, fast, reliable, and efficient communication and information storage system. It evolved to miniaturize and centralize the nervous system. If it did not, then each nerve in our body would have to be a least 50 times its current diameter. In order for the human nervous system to accomplish the same complexity our bodies would have to be enormous.

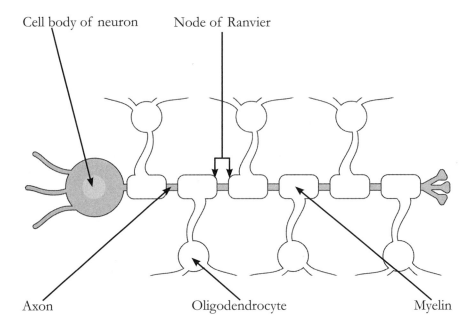

Figure 11.3. Nodes of Ranvier. Side view of a neuron, axon, myelin, and oligodendrocytes.

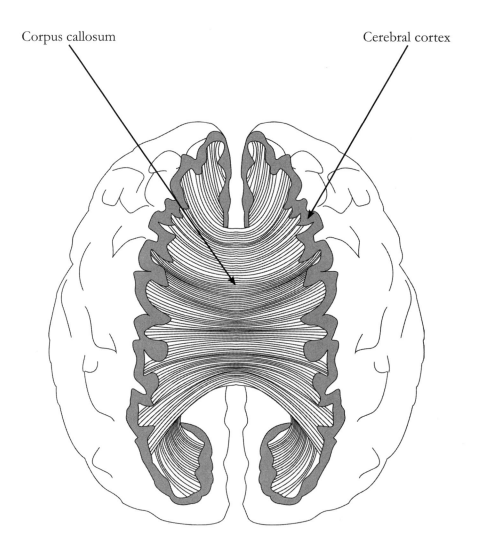

Figure 11.4. The corpus callosum. Top view of the brain. A portion of the cerebral cortex has been removed to show an example of one of the largest myelinated axon tracts (substantia alba) called the "corpus callosum."

Myelin disturbance

What happens when myelin does not form properly or breaks down? Neural communication is disturbed because the electrochemical current (action potential) traveling along axons is disrupted.

Neural communication is network communication: many thousands of neurons are involved each neural process. Every neuron in a network can receive, integrate, store, and send information. Neural work is built into the design of a neuron: its dendrites receive, its cell body integrates and stores, and its axon sends.

A neuron is intricately designed to transmit signals. Four aspects of neural signaling design are dedicated to: information processing, processing speed, signaling speed, and exquisite precision in the timing of signals. This design allows neurons to signal throughout an entire network with coordinated, exact timing.

Myelin is involved in the speed and timing of neural communication. Action potential speed (APS) increases when either the diameter of an axon increases or the amount of myelin wrapped around the axon increases. APS is important because the nervous system needs to receive information and react quickly. Timing is essential because thousands of signals converge upon, or diverge from, specific neural nodes quicker than the blink of an eye. When signals reaching or leaving nodes are not timed precisely, networks breakdown.

Breakdown of signaling can cause many problems. A partial list follows: autism spectrum disorders, difficulty concentrating, memory or cognitive impairment, motor impairment, multiple sclerosis, mood disorders, leukodystrophy, cerebral palsy, developmental delays, post-concussion syndrome, or pain.

CNS myelin is made of oligodendrocyte cell membrane wrapped tightly around a section of an axon. One oligodendrocyte myelinates about 50 different axons. Many oligodendrocytes myelinate each axon. The ability of oligodendrocytes to produce, maintain, and heal myelin can become disrupted. Disruption can be due to many factors, such as CNS infection, toxicity, blood flow disruption, interstitial fluid congestion, and biomechanical stressors that arise within the parenchyma or migrate through the pia-glial interface.

Craniosacral therapy corrective techniques can reach oligodendrocytes through the pia-glial interface because oligodendrocytes and myelin are surrounded by, and in some instances interconnected with, astrocytes. The astrocyte matrix can function as a myelin and oligodendrocyte corrective interface, which extends the reach of a craniosacral therapy practitioner's hands all the way from bone into the deepest regions of the CNS substantia alba (myelin and axons).

Chapter 12

Microglia, microgliosis, and astrogliosis

When glial cells undergo reactive changes in response to infection, toxicity or damage within the central nervous system (CNS), the glial reaction is called "gliosis." There are two forms of gliosis:
- microgliosis, and
- astrogliosis.

In this chapter microglial cells are described first, followed by a discussion of both forms of gliosis.

Microglia

Microglia are the immune cells of the CNS. They are derived from non-neural tube cells, called "embryonic mesoderm." Microglia become part of the CNS before the blood-brain barrier forms and before the embryonic neural tube transformation into primitive CNS structures is complete. Microglia have the highest cell division rate of any glial cell.

Micro-domains

Microglia are evenly distributed throughout the CNS so that each cell has its own individual section of three-dimensional space (Figure 12.1). They do not form interconnections as other glia do, such as astrocyte-to-oligodendrocyte or astrocyte-to-astrocyte interconnections. This is because microglia must be free to move within the CNS parenchyma when mounting an immune response.

Microglial receptors

Microglia have many receptors that can monitor the activity of cells and the cell environment for signs of damage, debris, infection, or other stressors (Figure 12.2). Among these are "pattern-recognition receptors," whose function is to detect invading pathogens such as bacteria and viruses. Microglia also have receptors for neurotransmitters, neuromodulators, and neurohormones. They have many ion channels. Microglia have receptors for immune-signaling molecules and proteins, called "cytokines" or "chemokines," as well as channels through which they secrete cytokines and chemokines to signal to other microglia, astrocytes, and neurons.

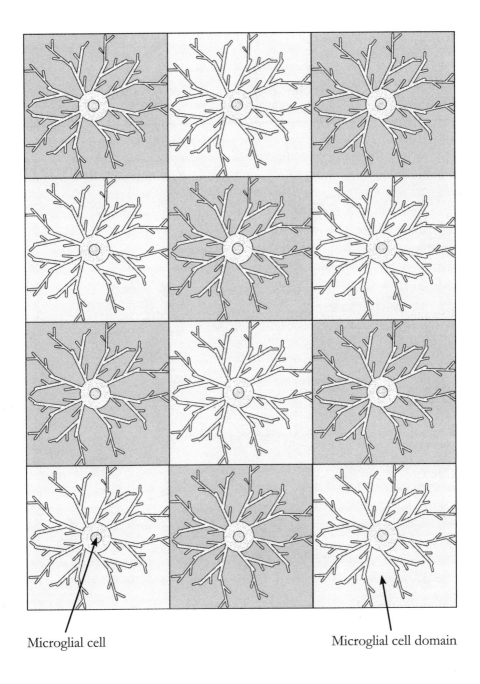

Figure 12.1. Mircoglial domains.

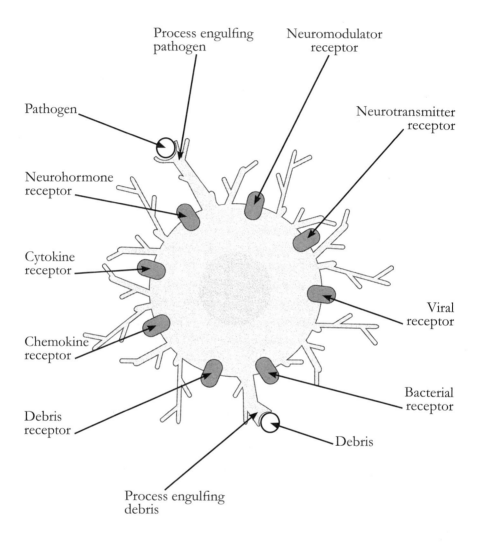

Figure 12.2. Microglial receptors. Microglia have an array of receptors, some of which are shown in the figure above. Also shown are microglial processes engulfing harmful substances.

Microglial activity must be precisely controlled in order to clear tissue and fluid of debris, toxins, or other harmful agents; while at the same time, they must protect delicate neural circuits and glia from harm. The wide array of microglial receptors allows microglia to precisely regulate their activity in relationship to the level of challenge in a specific CNS region. Also, microglia must modulate their level of response to produce the greatest benefit and least amount of harm.

Microglial states

Microglia can take on three different states, which are called:
- "resting," the normal surveillance state, considered a non-pathological reactive state;
- "activated," a pathological reactive state when they appear as rounded phagocytic cells; and
- "dystrophic," a period of decline and deterioration.

Resting microglial state

During the resting state cell bodies of microglia remain stationary while their processes scan their environment, which is called the "surveillance state." They do this by rotating back and forth while extending and contracting their processes. This resting state is not really resting at all but is an active and dynamic ongoing search for debris, pathogens, and cell stress (Figure 12.3).

Every speck of a microglial cell domain is scanned three to four times a day. Microglia search for metabolic waste and elements of deteriorated tissue. Once debris is found, microglia extend their processes to engulf the debris, which is then broken down into non-harmful elements within the microglial cell body (Figure 12.4).

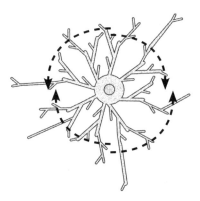

Figure 12.3. Resting state. Microglia scanning its domain for debris or pathogens.

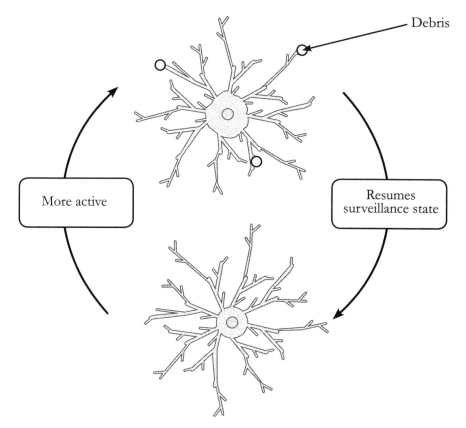

Figure 12.4. Resting state. Microglial cell becomes more active. After the harmful substance has been removed, it reverts back to its surveillance state.

Activated microglial phase

The microglial activated phase is also known as "microgliosis." When microglia sense CNS pathological states, such as infection, tissue injury, or harmful protein accumulation, they respond in a number of ways. The typical response is to:
- migrate to the site of pathology or damage;
- multiply to rapidly increase their number at the site;
- release immune-signaling cytokines and chemokines;
- initiate an inflammatory response and release pro-inflammatory factors, such as nitric oxide and Tumor Necrosis Factor, which help destroy and clear infectious agents;
- ingest (phagocytize) tissue debris and pathogens;
- degrade phagocytized elements;
- send fragments of pathogens, called "antigens," to peripheral immune cells by way of the vascular system; and
- modulate microglial response to meet the severity and nature of tissue pathology (Figure 12.5).

Dystrophic microglial phase

It is important to note that phagocytosis by microglial cells is ongoing; it does not only occur during the activated phase. Whenever microglia find debris during their resting state, they engulf then degrade it; however, they do not switch to an activated phase unless it is necessary. In this way, resting microglia keep their micro-domains clear of waste, dead cells, and tissue debris without an excessive response (Figure 12.6).

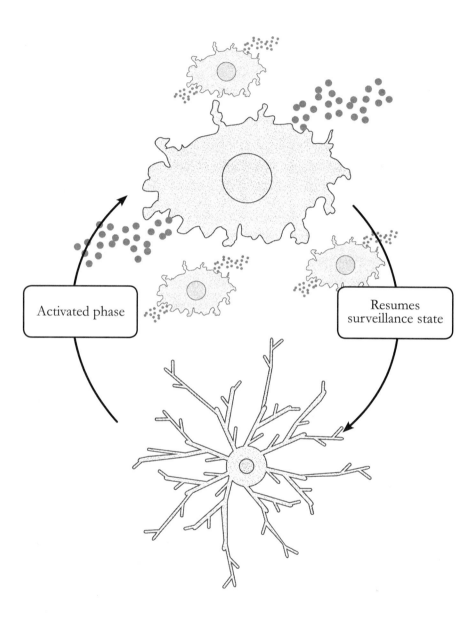

Figure 12.5. Activated state. Microglial cell transforms into the activated phase and then will revert back to its surveillance state once the harmful substance has been removed.

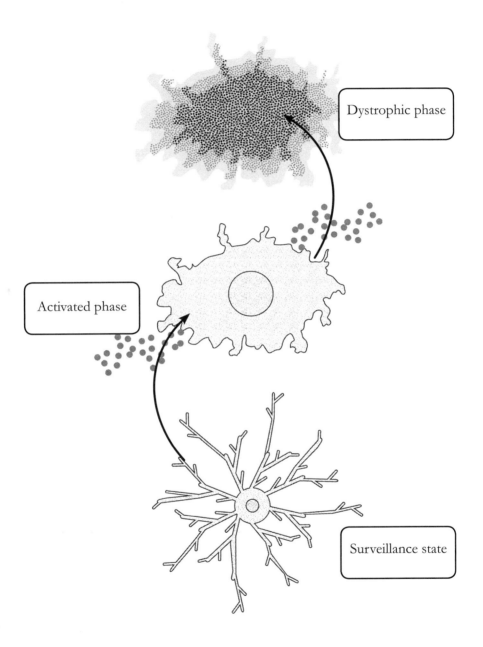

Figure 12.6. Dystrophic state. Microglia becomes activated and if no longer needed or no longer functional, it will degrade.

Microglia and neural plasticity

Dying neurons signal to microglia, and microglia respond by removing the neuron debris. This process is also used when synapses and dendrites are no longer of use: neurons signal to microglia so microglia can remove (strip) synapses and dendrites. This is an integral part of neural plasticity. Myelin waste is cleared in the same way, which is essential because myelin molecules at an injury site inhibit axonal outgrowth and remyelination. In this way, microglia are involved in helping to shape and maintain neurological networks throughout life. This process usually occurs without microglia taking on an activated state.

Microglia help heal the CNS

Microglia secrete proteins that help heal and protect neurons and capillaries, such as:
- "brain-derived neurotrophic factor" that helps support existing neurons and encourages the growth of new neurons and synapses,
- "nerve growth factor" that encourages the growth and survival of neurons,
- "basic fibroblast growth factor" that may help repair blood vessels and repair the BBB after BBB damage, and
- "glial cell-derived neurotrophic factor" that helps support neuron survival.

Microglia and synapse formation

During CNS development, astrocytes are the primary cells that produce and secrete extracellular proteins called "thrombospondins" (TSPs).

TSPs induce synaptic formation, called "synaptogenesis." Microglia also participate in the very early stages of synaptogenesis and neural network formation by secreting TSPs.

Astrogliosis

When astrocytes respond to CNS insult it is called "astrogliosis." This response is graded to meet the level of damage or infection.

There are three levels of astrogliosis:
- mild,
- moderate, and
- severe.

There are two forms of severe astrogliosis:
- diffuse astrogliosis, and
- reactive astrogliosis with compact scar.

Astrocytes lose their typical domain organization in both of the severe forms. Astrocytes maintain their typical domain organization in the mild and moderate forms (Figure 12.7).

Mild astrogliosis

Astrocytes remove local cell debris and pathogens as part of their normal housekeeping chores by extending processes that attach to the debris and pull it to the cell body to be engulfed. This is one of the mildest forms of astrogliosis. Astrocytes may hypertrophy slightly during this phase. They revert back to their typical shape when the engulfed debris has broken down. During this process astrocytes maintain their typical domain organization (Figure 12.8).

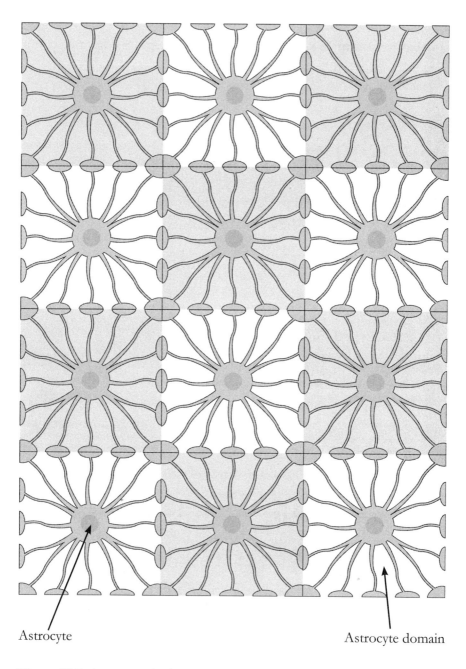

Astrocyte   Astrocyte domain

Figure 12.7. Astrocytes in their typical non-overlapping domain organization throughout the CNS.

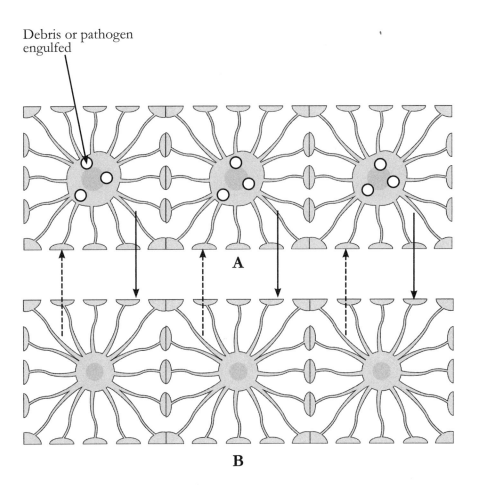

Figure 12.8. Mild astrogliosis. **A:** Astrocytes may hypertrophy slightly during this phase (dashed arrows). **B:** Astrocytes revert back to their typical shape (solid arrows).

Moderate astrogliosis

In moderate forms of astrogliosis, astrocytes hypertrophy from engulfing debris or pathogens, but they do not lose their normal astrocyte domain pattern, nor do they proliferate. This form of astrogliosis is usually in response to mild trauma, mild immune response, or in areas distant from CNS lesions. Once the insult is resolved, the astrocytes return to their healthy tissue state, and there is little or no long-term effect (Figure 12.9).

Diffuse astrogliosis

One severe form of astrogliosis is called "diffuse astrogliosis." It results in long-lasting or permanent changes in CNS architecture due to astrocyte hypertrophy, astrocyte proliferation, loss of astrocyte domains, and interlocking and overlapping of astrocytes. These changes can extend over large areas of the CNS. The cause of this astrocyte response is due to a higher degree of damage than in the mild or moderate forms of astrogliosis. This type of astrogliosis can lead to long-term ill effects (Figure 12.10).

Reactive astrogliosis with compact glial scar

Another severe form of astrogliosis is called "reactive astrogliosis with compact glial scar." This is a similar reaction to the "diffuse" form; however, in this form there is a high level of proliferation, overlapping, and interlocking of astrocytes that creates a compact border known as a "compact glial scar" (Figure 12.11).

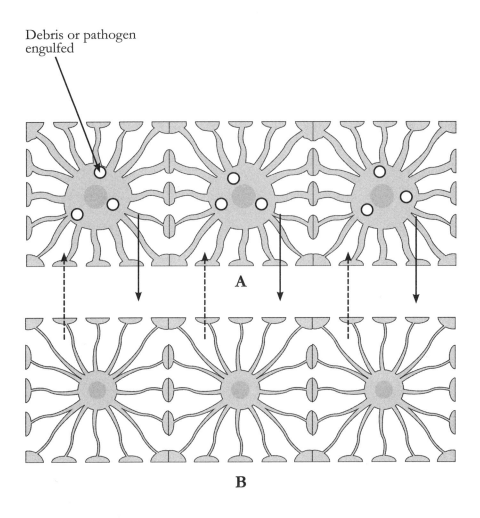

Figure 12.9. Moderate astrogliosis. **A:** Astrocytes hypertrophy during this phase (dashed arrows). **B:** Astrocytes revert back to their typical shape (solid arrows).

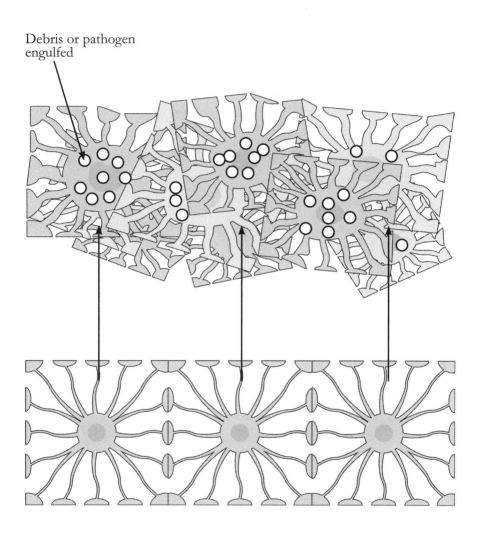

Figure 12.10. Diffuse astrogliosis. Astrocytes hypertrophy, proliferate, and lose domain organization during this phase (solid arrows). Astrocytes are unable to return to their typical form.

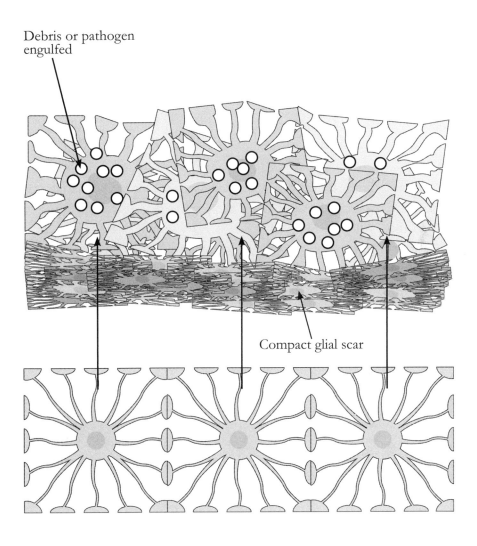

Figure 12.11. Severe reactive astrogliosis with compact scar. Astrocytes hypertrophy, proliferate, lose domain organization, and form a compact glial scar during this phase (solid arrows). Astrocytes are unable to return to their typical form.

Compact glial scars contain substances, such as myelin fragments, that inhibit both axon growth and cell migration. These scars are usually permanent and continue even when the insult has resolved. Glial scars dramatically alter CNS architecture.

Some of the causes of compact glial scar formation, which is the most severe from of astrogliosis, are severe tissue damage (trauma), necrosis, infection, infiltration of autoimmune inflammatory elements, CNS autoimmune disease, and viral or bacterial infection (Figure 12.12).

One very important function of glial scars is to encircle a pathological area and then attract and instruct inflammatory cells. This helps to isolate areas when an intense inflammatory response is needed, and it helps to minimize the effect upon surrounding tissue (Figure 12.13 and Figure 12.14) .

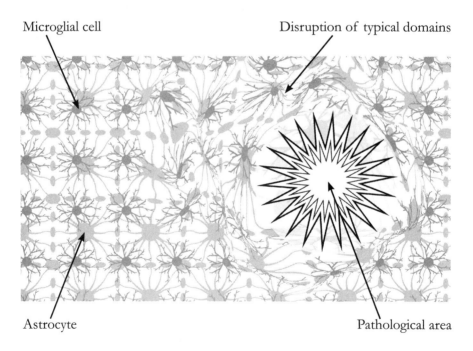

Figure 12.12. Disturbance of astrocyte and microglial domains due to pathology, such as: trauma, infection, debris, toxin, or stroke.

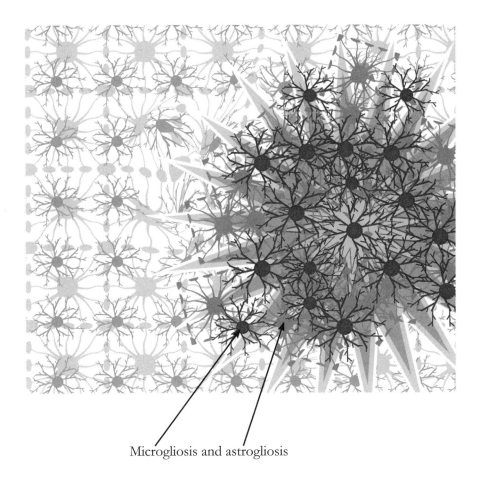

Microgliosis and astrogliosis

Figure 12.13. Microgliosis and astrogliosis. Microglia and astrocytes lose their typical domain organization, proliferate, and migrate to the site of pathology.

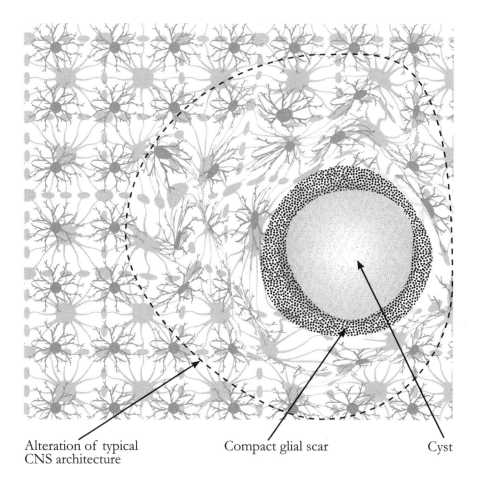

Figure 12.14. Compact glial scar. Area within the dashed line shows the disruption of CNS architecture due to the initial pathological state and the compact glial scar.

When microglial or astrocyte processes go awry

Microglia and astrocytes perform critical functions, some of which are:
- forming synapses,
- stripping synapses,
- protecting the CNS from infection or toxicity,
- breaking down and clearing debris,
- secreting substances to heal CNS tissue damage, and
- forming glial scars to isolate damaged CNS tissue.

There are times when these functions become disrupted leading to pathology. For example, both microglia and astrocytes monitor synapse activity. When neurons stop sending signals at axon terminal synapses, or no longer receive signals at dendritic spine synapses, then three things will take place:
- microglia converge upon the synapse and secrete substances that break down the synapse (known as "synaptic stripping" or "synaptic pruning"),
- microglia and astrocytes will take in and then degrade synapse fragments, and
- astrocyte end-feet seal off the area.

If the neuron tries repeatedly signaling at the stripped terminal synapse or receives input at the stripped dendritic spine synapse, astrocyte end-feet pull away from the synaptic area so the synapse can reform.

If microglial stripping is unregulated, then too many synapses will be stripped or synapses will not form. If astrocyte sealing of synaptic areas is unchecked, then synapses will not form.

When microglial cell activity or astrocyte processes become distorted, a host of pathological changes may occur. A partial list follows: CNS infection, CNS inflammation, Alzheimer's disease, Parkinson's disease, atypical brain development, autism spectrum disorder, chronic pain, or cognitive dysfunction.

Dysregulation of microglia or astrocytes can occur in response to being overly burdened by infection, toxicity, debris, or tissue damage. If any of the glial barriers or the blood-brain barrier break down, then infection, toxicity, or injurious substances can enter the interstitium. Also, interstitial tissue damage can take place due to barrier disruption.

I will use mild head trauma and subsequent gliosis as an example of how meningeal stress can lead to gliosis. Research has shown that even mild trauma to the skull can cause a breakdown of the pia mater membrane and outer glial limiting membrane in the area adjacent to the injury. Then microglia rush to the area, proliferate, and mount a response. Astrocytes also mount a response and proliferate.

If the pia mater membrane or outer glial membrane cannot heal quickly, an ongoing state of microgliosis and astrogliosis persists in the area. This causes chronic cerebral inflammation that can lead to excessive cell pressure, cell death, debris buildup, or interstitial fluid congestion. One or more of these stressors can cause mild to severe cognitive dysfunction or motor impairment, especially if the pia mater membrane or outer glial membrane does not heal.

Craniosacral therapy (CST) techniques can lessen both meningeal adverse strain and outer glial limiting membrane stress that was caused by the trauma. Decreasing these stressors can bolster healing of the pia mater membrane and outer glial limiting membrane. In response to healing, barrier form and function can be reestablished, and interstitial stressors can be cleansed from the area. As the interstitium is cleansed of debris and irritants, then microglia resume their resting state and astrocytes resume their typical state. Also, both microglia and astrocytes secrete substances that help to heal damaged neurons and heal the blood-brain barrier.

This is one example of how biomechanical stress can lead to microgliosis and astrogliosis. There are many other causes of gliosis that, fortunately, CST techniques can reach and help to correct through the pia-glial interface and its interconnection with the entire CNS parenchyma.

Chapter 13

Retinal glia

*G*lia are essential components of the eye. In this chapter the basic structures of the eye will be discussed first, followed by a discussion of glial cells within the retina.

The eye has two basic parts. The "optical" part collects light and projects it onto the retina. The retina is the "neural" part: it converts light into neural signals that are sent to various brain regions for processing. The retina is part of the central nervous system because it originates from an outcropping of the neural tube. Retinal neurons and their complex processes are aided by, and rely upon, retinal glia. The predominate type of glial cell found in the retina is called the Muller cell (Figure 13.1).

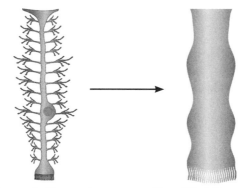

Schematic illustration   Simplified illustration

Figure 13.1. Muller cell.

The eye projects light upon the retina (Figure 13.2). Light-sensitive cells of the retina, called "photoreceptors," receive light and convert it into neural signals (Figure 13.3). These signals are conveyed to a series of neurons within the retina for integration and then relayed by way of the optic nerve to several brain regions, resulting in visual perception.

"Rods" and "cones" are the photoreceptor cells of the retina. There are an average of 4.6 million cones (used for bright light, color reception, and detailed vision) and 92 million rods (used for low light vision).

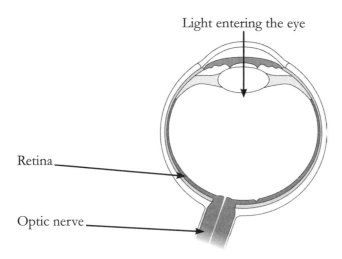

Figure 13.2. The eye (cross section).

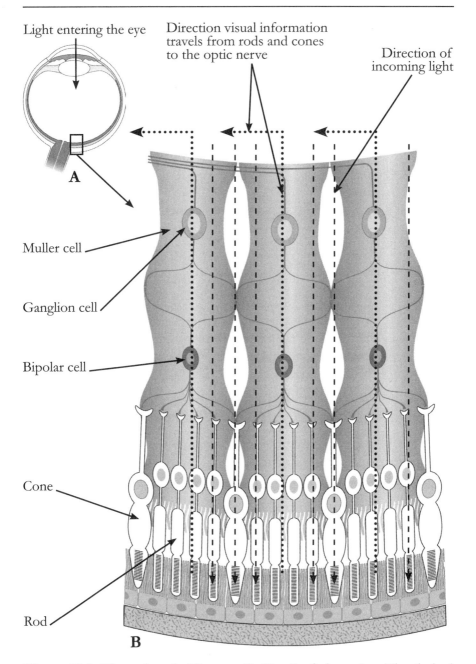

Figure 13.3. The retina. **A:** The eye. **B:** Detail of the retina. The dashed line shows light passing through retinal cells as it travels to rods and cones (photoreceptor cells). The dotted line shows the direction visual information is transmitted from rods and cones towards the optic nerve.

Glia within the retina

There are four types of glial cells found in the retina. They are covered in the following sections:
- Muller cells,
- retinal astrocytes,
- retinal microglia, and
- retinal pigment epithelial cells.

Muller cells

Muller cells, specialized astrocyte-like cells, are the most abundant glial cells of the retina: they span almost the entire retinal thickness. They are spaced regularly throughout the retina, forming micro-domains, similar to the way each astrocyte within the brain has an individual non-overlapping area. Each Muller cell surrounds the neurons, axons, and blood vessels in its particular area.

Some of the crucial roles Muller cells fulfill are the following:
- provide nutritive (trophic) substances to neurons;
- remove metabolic waste products;
- regulate the volume of the extracellular space;
- control ion concentrations, such as potassium, through uptake of ions or spatial buffering;
- regulate water flow;
- help maintain the blood-retina barrier and retinal blood flow;
- release gliotransmitters and other neuroactive substances, thereby modulating neural activity;
- take up neurotransmitter from the synaptic cleft and recycle it;
- provide neurotransmitter precursors to neurons, such as glutamine;
- supply energy substrates to neurons;
- modulate the immune and inflammatory response within the eye;
- help buffer biomechanical deformations of retinal tissue;

- maintain optimal pH balance;
- respond to neural signaling with intracellular calcium waves that may act as an intracellular signaling system; and
- supply glutathione, which protects both neurons and glia from oxidative injury.

Muller cells also appear to transmit light. Photoreceptors receive light after it has passed through other retinal cells. A surprisingly small degree of image distortion takes place considering light tends to scatter when passing through varying layers of cells. Muller cells have been shown to function as optical fibers that guide light to photoreceptors with minimal image distortion. They span the retinal space from where light enters the retina all the way to photoreceptor cells. The structure of Muller cells and their arrangement within the retina make them excellent light collectors and light transmitters (Figure 13.4).

Retinal microglia

Retinal microglia are resident retinal immune cells. They function the same way as microglia within the brain by:
- cleansing the tissue of debris, bacteria, or viruses;
- initiating an inflammatory response as needed;
- replicating and migrating throughout the entire retina when necessary; and
- secreting tissue-repair substances.

Retinal astrocytes

Retinal astrocytes are found within a few layers of the retina where they wrap around blood vessels, neurons, and axons. They help regulate blood flow and buffer ion concentrations within their areas and appear to have many of the same functions as astrocytes within the brain and spinal cord.

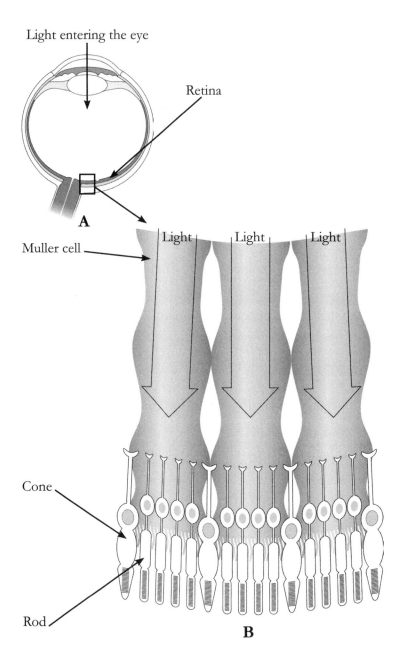

Figure 13.4. Muller cells transmit light. **A:** The eye. **B:** Detail of Muller cells transmitting light. Arrows show light traveling within Muller cells toward photoreceptors.

Retinal pigment epithelium

The outer part of the retina is composed of specialized glial cells that create the retinal pigment epithelium (RPE). The RPE cells have long microvilli in which photoreceptors are embedded. A primary and essential function of the RPE is to engulf and destroy (phagocytize) debris created by photoreceptors. It is estimated that each photoreceptor cell sheds and renews 10 percent of its volume per day in order to decrease photo-oxidative stress. The RPE must constantly process and dispose of photoreceptor debris (Figure 13.5).

The RPE is responsible for:
- supplying neuroprotective elements, growth factors, and immune substances;
- absorbing light that is not absorbed by photoreceptors in order to limit image distortion and limit oxidative stress;
- supporting the blood-retina barrier between the choroid and the retina; and
- helping control the flow of nutrients, ions, waste products, and other molecules between the choroid and retina.

Craniosacral therapy can improve eye health

The eye can be regarded as a multi-layered ball of highly specialized tissue that is encased almost entirely within a protective fascial covering (the sclera). The sclera is continuous with the dura mater membrane encasing the optic nerve. Six extrinsic eye muscles controlling eye movement attach to the eye. Intrinsic eye muscles control the lens and pupil. The eye is suspended in a pocket of adipose tissue that is tucked into the bony orbit. The bony orbit has foramina within it through which pass vessels and nerves into and out of the brain. Eyelids protect the front of the eye.

Fascial adverse strain can overly stress any of the eye's specialized layers, eye muscles, orbital fat and bone, or eyelids. This stress can alter vision by: deforming the shape of the eye, causing fluid congestion and pressure within the eye, or distorting the structure of the retina. Also, the nerve that transmits visual information to the brain from the eye (optic nerve) can be twisted, pulled, or compressed by fascial distortions. Meningeal stress can also harm the optic nerve.

A meningeal tube called the "meningeal sheath" encases the optic nerve. As the optic nerve enters the orbit from the brain the meningeal sheath blends with the fascial sheath of the eyeball. Adverse meningeal stress can compress, twist, or pull either the optic nerve or the retina. This structural distortion can cause problems such as astigmatism, myopia, presbyopia, or dry eyes.

Craniosacral therapy techniques can lessen distortion patterns of bone, muscle, fascia related to the eye, eye structures, or the optic nerve meningeal sheath. Decreasing these distortions can help the eye reform itself, decrease stress of the optic nerve, and improve retinal shape. As the form of the eye improves then light can be transmitted to the retina efficiently, and visual information can be transmitted by the optic nerve to brain regions most effectively. Also, reformation of the retina can improve the retina's ability to receive, integrate and send visual information. These improvements often lead to improved eyesight.

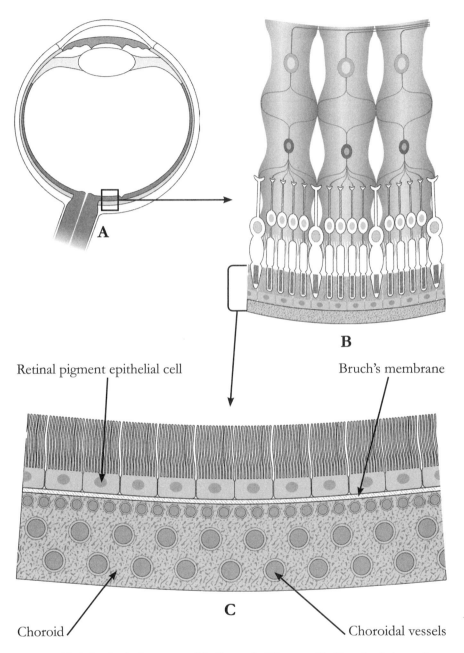

Figure 13.5. Retinal pigment epithelium. **A:** The eye. **B:** Detail of the retina. **C:** Detail of the retinal pigment epithelium (RPE) and the choroid. The choroid is a bed of highly vascular tissue encasing the RPE.

Chapter 14

Peripheral nervous system glia

*T*his chapter describes glia of the peripheral nervous system (PNS). PNS glial research is lagging behind central nervous system (CNS) glial research. Yet, the use of PNS glia during craniosacral therapy can be very effective in reducing PNS dysfunction. PNS glia are presented in the following sections:
- Schwann cells,
- sympathetic and parasympathetic satellite glia,
- enteric glia,
- sensory system satellite glia,
- common satellite glial cell functions, and
- olfactory ensheathing glia.

Peripheral neurons and glia are generated by neural crest cells (Figure 14.1). Neural crest cells originate from an embryonic cell layer, called the "ectoderm," and travel throughout the embryo to become many different cell types.

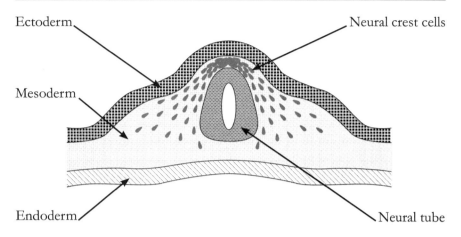

Figure 14.1. Transverse section of a 24-day-old embryo. The ectoderm, mesoderm, and endoderm are the three embryonic cell layers. Neural crest cells and the neural tube originate from the ectoderm. Refer to Chapter 6, "Radial glia and central nervous system development."

Schwann cells

There are three types of Schwann cells:
- myelinating Schwann cells,
- non-myelinating Schwann cells, and
- terminal Schwann cells, also known as "perisynaptic Schwann cells."

Myelinating Schwann cells

Myelinating Schwann cells insulate individual axon sections. Axons of the PNS are myelinated like axons within the CNS: sections of myelin, called "internodes," encase the length of an axon; and tiny gaps between internodes, called "nodes of Ranvier," separate internodes (Figure 14.2 and Figure 14.3).

One internode is myelinated by a single Schwann cell. Myelinating Schwann cells function like oligodendrocytes in the CNS by speeding up and helping to organize neural signaling.

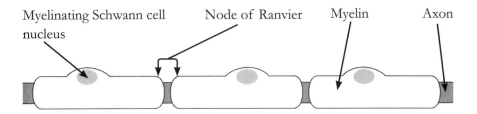

Figure 14.2. Side view of three myelinating Schwann cells.

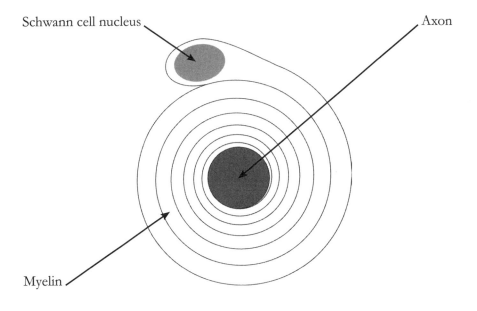

Figure 14.3. Transverse section of a myelinating Schwann cell.

Potassium regulation at nodes of Ranvier

The amount of potassium increases within nodes of Ranvier when neurons signal. If too much potassium builds up, then chaotic neural signaling, or shutting down of signaling, can take place. Regulating the amount of potassium within nodes of Ranvier is a crucial function of Schwann cells.

Schwann cell potassium regulation

Schwann cell extensions, called "Schwann cell perinodal microvilli," project into nodes of Ranvier (Figure 14.4). Microvilli are thin hairlike microscopic cell membrane extensions. Perinodal microvilli have potassium channels within their cell membrane through which excess potassium travels into the Schwann cell. This potassium will then flow through a thin connective tissue layer surrounding the Schwann cell, called the "basal lamina," to enter the surrounding space and be absorbed by either the lymphatic system or venous system.

Non-myelinating Schwann cells

Non-myelinating Schwann cells encase small diameter unmyelinated axons, like those conveying sensations of pain, temperature, touch, itch, and pressure. Non-myelinating Schwann cells adjoin one another tightly without forming nodes of Ranvier (Figure 14.5 and Figure 14.6).

Perisynaptic Schwann cells

Perisynaptic Schwann cells encase neuromuscular junctions (synapses) (Figure 14.7); they are essential for synapse development, signaling, maintenance, regeneration, and the recovery of nerve function after injury.

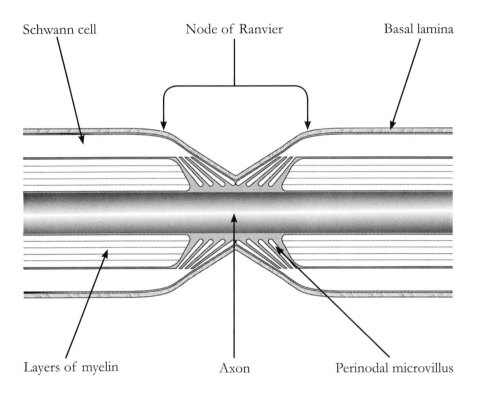

Figure 14.4. Schwann cell perinodal microvilli.

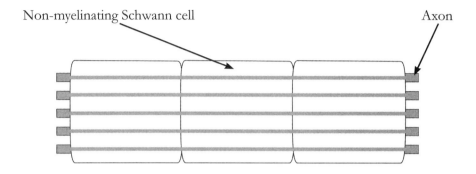

Figure 14.5. Side view of three non-myelinating Schwann cells.

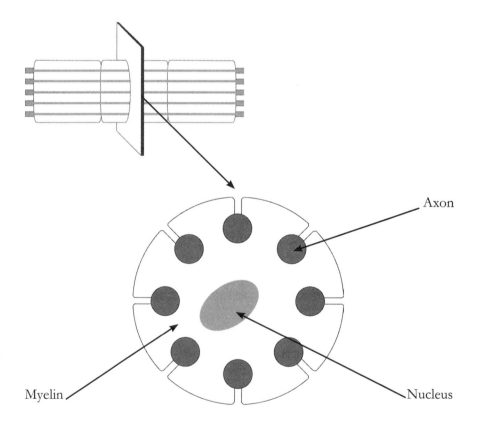

Figure 14.6. Transverse section of a non-myelinating Schwann cell.

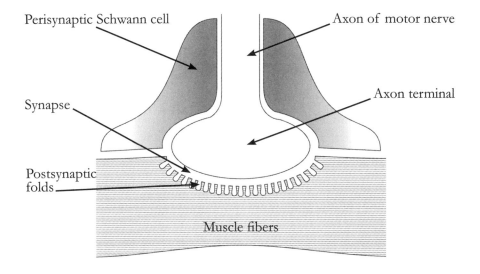

Figure 14.7. Cross section of a neuromuscular junction with perisynaptic Schwann cells.

Wallerian degeneration

Schwann cells assist in regeneration and remyelination of damaged PNS axons. Axons may degenerate due to damage caused by trauma, infection, inflammation, demyelination, or cell stress. Axon degeneration distal to a lesion is called "Wallerian degeneration."

PNS Wallerian degeneration

PNS Wallerian degeneration occurs in the following sequence (Figure 14.8):
- demyelination of the damaged axon distal to the lesion,
- degeneration of the axon and its myelin sheath,
- accumulation of myelin fragments and cell debris in the area,
- phagocytosis of debris from the surrounding tissue by Schwann cells and macrophages,
- proliferation of Schwann cells in the area,
- sprouting of the damaged axon and axon growth,
- secretion of growth factors by Schwann cells,
- secretion of guidance molecules by Schwann cells that help the axon reach its destination, and
- secretion of guidance molecules by perisynaptic Schwann cells that help to reform the neuromuscular junction.

CNS Wallerian degeneration

CNS Wallerian degeneration occurs in the following sequence (Figure 14.9):
- demyelination of the damaged axon distal to the lesion,
- degeneration of the axon and its myelin sheath,
- accumulation of myelin fragments and cell debris in the area,
- activation of microglia (microgliosis) to clear debris,
- activation of astrocytes (astrogliosis) to clear debris and to limit spreading of damage to other areas of the CNS,
- formation of a compact glia scar that isolates the damaged area from surrounding tissue,
- axon regeneration is blocked by the glial scar, and
- neuron and axon may eventually degenerate if the neuron is unable to reform synaptic connections.

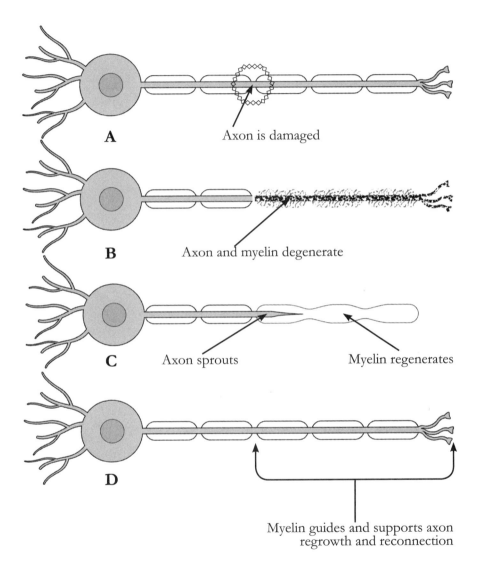

Figure 14.8. Peripheral nervous system response to Wallerian degeneration. The order of the process is from **A** to **D**.

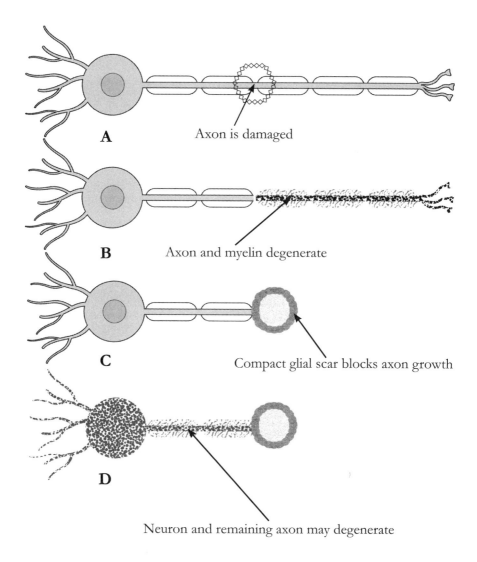

Figure 14.9. Central nervous system response to Wallerian degeneration. The order of the process is from **A** to **D**.

Sympathetic and parasympathetic division satellite glia

Through the innervation of glands, cardiac muscle, and smooth muscle, the autonomic nervous system (ANS) regulates involuntary body functions, such as digestion, heartbeat, blood flow, and breathing. The ANS consists of three divisions:
- sympathetic division, also known as the "freeze, fight, flight, fright, or faint" division;
- parasympathetic division, also known as the "rest, digest, or renew" division; and
- enteric division, also known as the "gut" division.

Glial cells are components of all three divisions of the ANS. Sympathetic and parasympathetic division satellite glia are discussed first, followed by a discussion of enteric glia.

Both sympathetic and parasympathetic divisions of the autonomic nervous system have ganglia located within their neurological networks (Figure 14.10 to Figure 14.12). The ganglia function as signal relay and neural integrative centers. Each ganglion is a cluster of neuronal cell bodies, axons, synapses, glial cells, blood vessels, and connective tissue. Glia within both sympathetic and parasympathetic ganglia are astrocyte-like cells called "satellite glial cells" (SGCs).

SGCs within each ganglion surround neurons (Figure 14.13 and Figure 14.14). The SGCs have numerous cell membrane channels and neurotransmitter receptors, form gap junctions, and function like CNS astrocytes. However, the structure of SGCs differs from that of astrocytes because SGCs do not:
- have cell processes,
- encase blood vessels, or
- form a ganglion-wide glial syncytium.

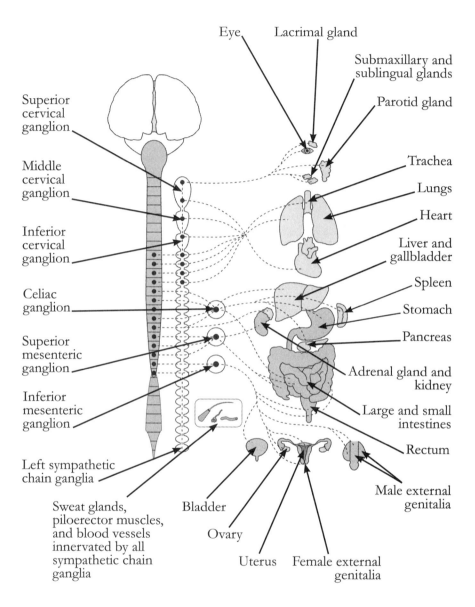

Figure 14.10. Anterior view of the sympathetic division of the autonomic nervous system showing the left sympathetic chain. The mid-line ganglia (celiac ganglion, superior mesenteric ganglion, and inferior mesenteric ganglion) are shown. They are offset from the mid-line to show the spinal cord levels (T1-L1) from which sympathetic nerves emerge.

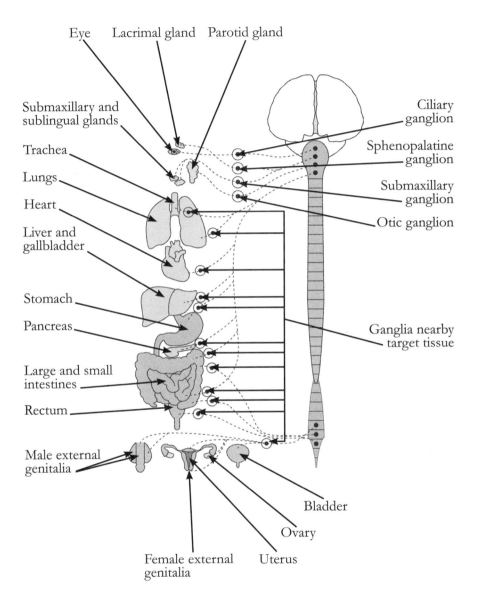

Figure 14.11. Anterior view of the parasympathetic division of the autonomic nervous system. The nerves emerge from the brainstem or sacral nerves S2-S4.

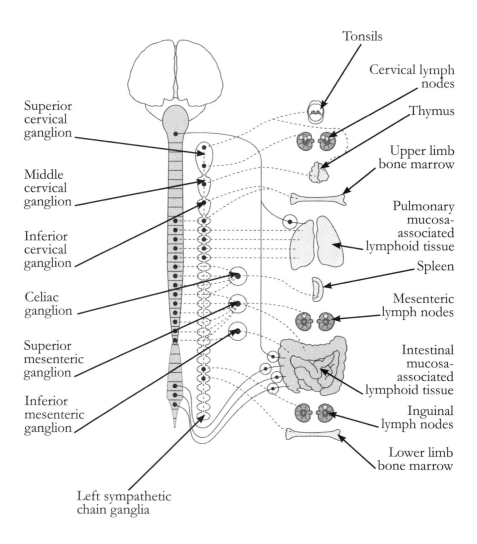

Figure 14.12. Sympathetic and parasympathetic innervation of immune organs. Anterior view of the left sympathetic chain and mid-line ganglia (celiac ganglion, superior mesenteric ganglion and inferior mesenteric ganglion) are shown. They are offset from the mid-line to show the spinal cord levels (T1-L1) from which sympathetic nerves emerge. Innervation of immune system organs shown as dashed lines). Anterior view of parasympathetic innervation of immune system organs. Innervation shown as solid lines.

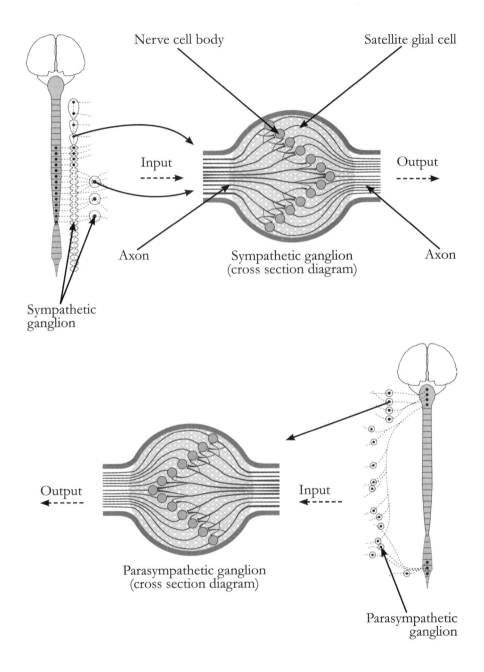

Figure 14.13. Diagram of sympathetic and parasympathetic ganglia.

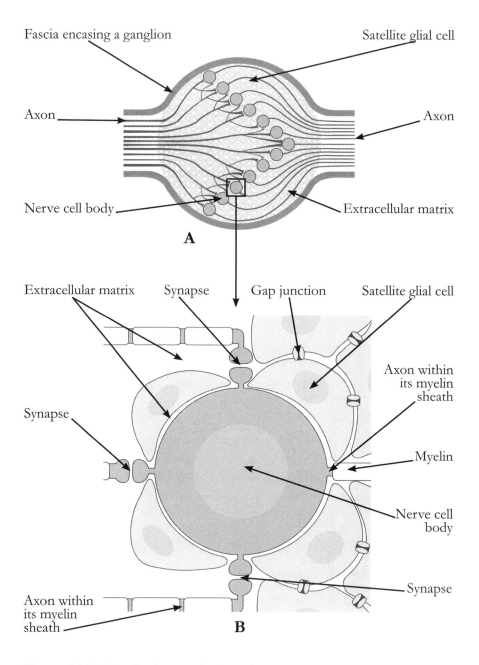

Figure 14.14. Detail of sympathetic and parasympathetic ganglia. **A:** Cross section diagram of a sympathetic or parasympathetic ganglion. **B:** Detail of satellite glia encasing a nerve cell body.

Enteric glia

The Enteric Nervous System (ENS) regulates both the digestive and absorptive processes of the gastrointestinal (GI) tract (Figure 14.15). The GI tract is vital for life because it is the organ in which food is broken down into essential nutrients that are then absorbed by the body. The breakdown of food takes place first in the mouth, then in the stomach, and then in the small intestine. Most of the nutrients from food are absorbed across the lining (epithelium) of the small intestine to then enter the body circulation. The large intestine primarily absorbs water through its epithelium. Undigested material and other waste products are excreted from the body at the lower end of the GI tract (the anus).

Toxins may be released when food is digested, or food may carry environmental irritants, parasites, or infectious agents, such as bacteria. The ENS controls immune protection against these harmful substances and controls the inflammatory response of the GI tract.

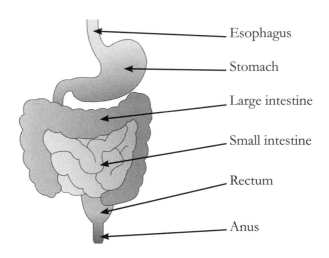

Figure 14.15. Gastrointestinal tract.

Glia within the GI tract are called "enteric glia." They are present throughout the entire GI tract. To date, research has focused primarily on two types of enteric glia: mucosal glia and glia within ENS ganglia. I will discuss enteric ganglia first.

Two continuous and interconnected neuroglial networks make up the ENS. These networks are called the "myenteric plexus" and the "submucosal plexus" (Figure 14.16). They are comprised of neurologically interconnected ganglia; each ganglion is tightly packed with neurons, axons, and glia. The myenteric plexus extends from the upper esophagus to the anal sphincter. The submucosal plexus is primarily found within the small and large intestines. There are approximately 100 million neurons in the ENS that form circuits directly controlling GI tract processes.

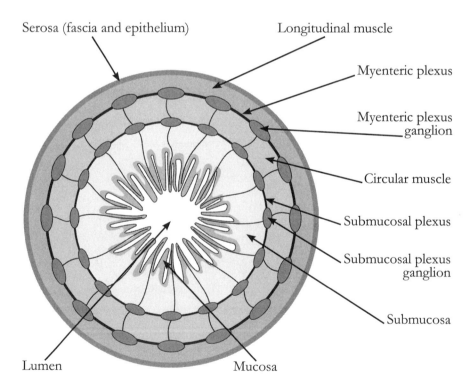

Figure 14.16. Cross section of the small intestine.

Enteric glial cell structure

Glia within ganglia of the ENS have an astrocyte-like form: they surround neurons and axons within enteric ganglia, and contact blood vessels, immune cells, and fibroblasts within the ganglia's connective tissue sheath (Figure 14.17 and Figure 14.18). Also, synapse-like junctions between enteric glia and enteric neurons have receptors for almost every gut neurotransmitter or neuromodulator.

Mucosal glia

Another type of enteric glial cell is called a "mucosal glial cell." It is found within the inner lining of the intestinal wall (mucosa); however, it is not contained within ganglia. Mucosal glia have a central body with many processes extending outward from it. These processes make contact with blood vessels, lymphatics, epithelial cells, and cells that are essential in mucosal healing, called "myofibroblasts." It appears that mucosal glia help manage mucosal structure, function, and healing through the integration and transfer of information among mucosal cells.

Enteric glial cell functions

Enteric glia have many critical functions, some of which are:
- protecting neurons and themselves by secreting trophic substances and antioxidants,
- integrating and regulating neurological signaling throughout the GI tract,
- modulating GI tract immune response,
- protecting and enhancing GI epithelial mucosa by secreting substances such as glutathione (s-nitrosoglutathione),
- regulating GI tract inflammation,

- responding to both sympathetic and parasympathetic innervation,
- integrating GI tract motion (peristalsis),
- regenerating enteric glia as needed, and
- modulating neural function through neuron-glia communication.

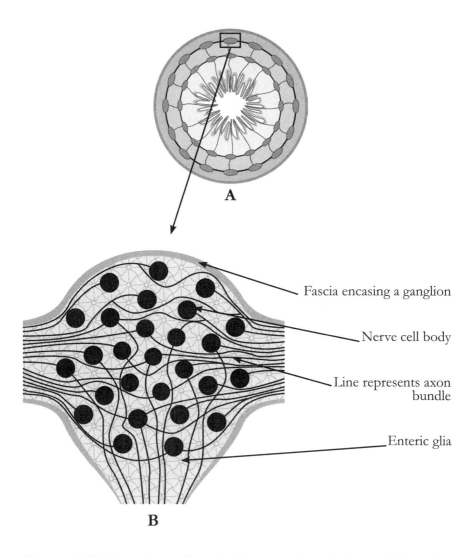

Figure 14.17. Enteric ganglion. **A:** Cross section of the small intestine. **B:** Cross section diagram of an enteric ganglion.

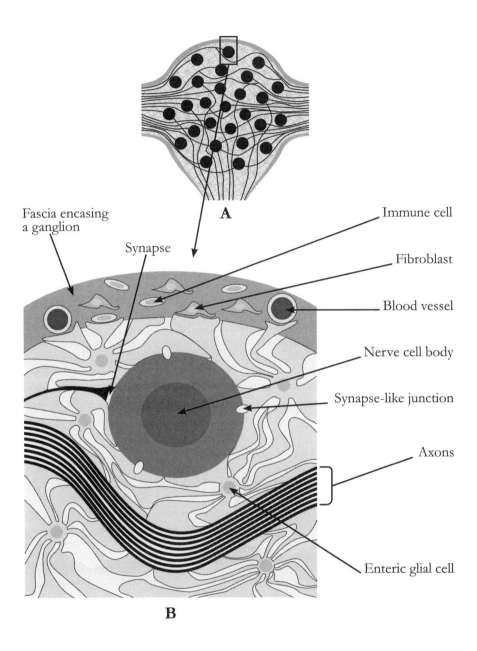

Figure 14.18. Enteric glia. **A:** Cross section diagram of an enteric ganglion. **B:** Detail diagram of enteric glia encasing neuronal cell body and axons. Enteric glia fill all the spaces in between neurons and axons within the ganglion.

Sensory system satellite glia

The sensory system processes sensory information such as touch, vision, hearing, smell, and taste. The "somatic sensory system" conveys sensations from the body to the CNS, such as heat, cold, touch, pressure, pain, limb position, and limb motion. Somatic sensory signals are transmitted to the CNS primarily by sensory nerves that have their nerve cell bodies within ganglia called "dorsal root ganglia" (DRG) (Figure 14.19 and Figure 14.20). These nerves each have an axon extending from its nerve cell body with one end (branch) of the axon extending into the periphery and one branch extending into the spinal cord (pseudounipolar nerve). DRG do not contain synapses.

Glial cells within DRG are called "satellite glia." Their form is similar to sympathetic and parasympathetic satellite glia (Figure 14.21 and Figure 4.22).

The other major sensory ganglia are the "trigeminal ganglia" and "nodose ganglia," both of which are structurally and functionally like DRG.

Common satellite glial cell functions

Satellite glial cells within sympathetic, parasympathetic, and DRG have similar functions, such as:
- controlling the micro-environment within the ganglia through the uptake, transport, and release of substances like neurotransmitters, neuromodulators, and potassium;
- supplying neurons with neurotransmitter substrates, such as glutamine; and
- removing debris or inflammatory substances.

CHAPTER 14 PERIPHERAL NERVOUS SYSTEM GLIA

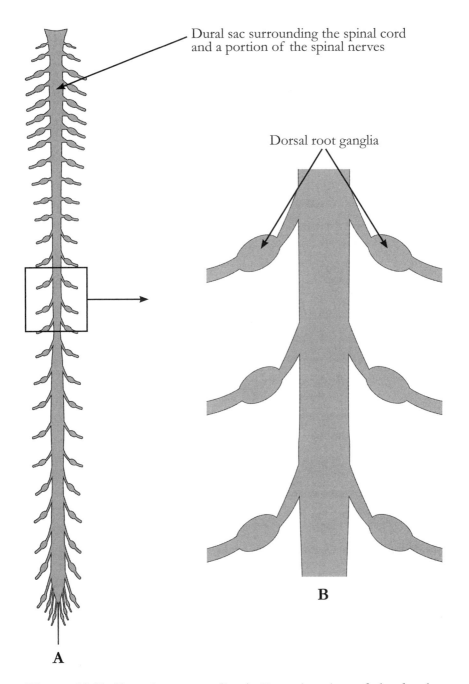

Figure 14.19. Dorsal root ganglia. **A:** Posterior view of the dural sac. **B:** Detail of the dural sac showing the location of dorsal root ganglia.

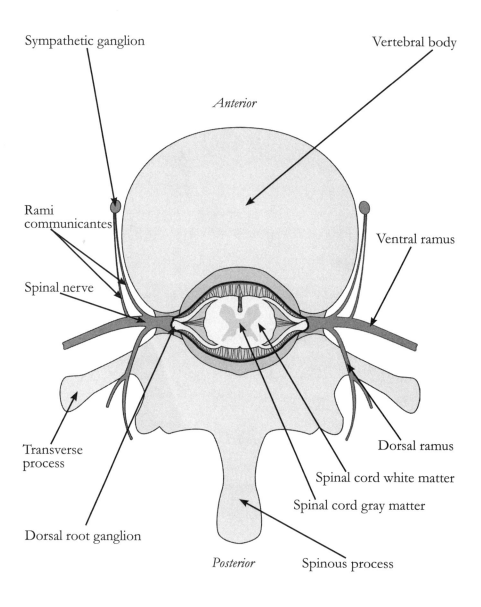

Figure 14.20. Transverse section of the vertebral column, spinal cord, and dorsal root ganglia.

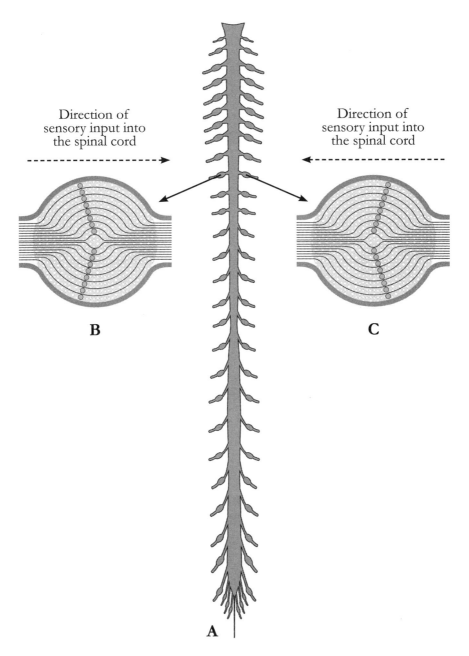

Figure 14.21. Dorsal root ganglia. **A:** Posterior view of the dural sac. **B:** Cross section detail of a left dorsal root ganglion. **C:** Cross section detail of a right dorsal root ganglion.

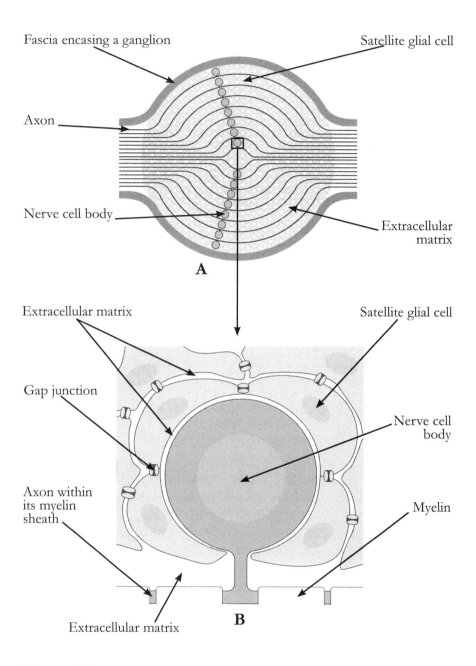

Figure 14.22. Dorsal root ganglion satellite glia. **A:** Cross section detail of a left dorsal root ganglion. **B:** Detail of satellite glia encasing a nerve cell body.

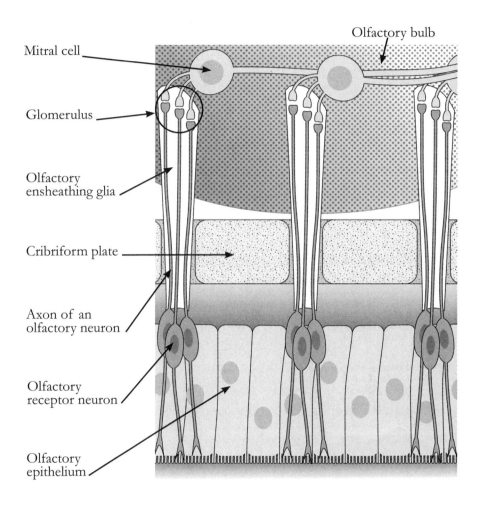

Figure 14.23. Olfactory nerves. Sagittal view of the cribriform plate and olfactory nerves. Olfactory receptor neurons send their axons through the cribriform plate of the ethmoid bone to synapse with "mitral cells" within "glomeruli." Olfactory glomeruli are found within the "olfactory bulb." Mitral cells relay signals to various brain regions, such as the amygdala and the insula.

Olfactory ensheathing glia

Olfactory receptor neurons extend their axons from the olfactory epithelium within the nasal cavity to reach the olfactory bulb within the cranial cavity. Olfactory receptor axons travel in small bundles encased within specialized glia called "olfactory ensheathing glia" (OEG) (Figure 14.23).

Olfactory neurons are renewed throughout life. Cells that will become new olfactory nerves, called "olfactory neural precursor cells," arise from the subventricular zone and then migrate to the olfactory bulb. This migration pathway is called the "rostral migratory stream." Diffused substances released by OEG help guide neural precursor cells along the rostral migratory stream, and they help regulate reproduction and specialization of olfactory cells.

To date little is known about OEG except for the functions listed above. OEG do not myelinate olfactory axons; however, experiments in rats have shown that when OEG are transplanted into a rat's demyelinated spinal cord, OEG promote remyelination. Also when OEG were transplanted into a rat's severely traumatized spinal cord, OEG facilitated axon growth and recovery of nerve function.

PNS glial dysfunction

PNS glial disturbance can cause a wide range of dysfunction. A partial list follows:
- damage to myelin can produce tingling and burning sensations (neuropathy), muscle weakness (hypotonia), loss of muscle control, muscle atrophy, or pain;
- injury to satellite glia within ANS ganglia can cause dizziness, fainting (syncope), excessive or decreased sweating, slow pupil

reaction, drooping eyelid, urinary incontinence, anxiety, difficulty sleeping, high blood pressure, erratic heart rate, constipation, dry mouth, or dry eyes;
- harm to satellite glia within DRG can cause chronic pain, spinal cord facilitated segments, spinal cord inflammation, imbalance, neuropathy, poor motor reflexes, or disturbed position-movement sensations (proprioceptive dysfunction);
- damage to enteric glia can cause intestinal pain, diarrhea or constipation, nausea, irritable bowel syndrome, reduced nutrient absorption, malnutrition, gastrointestinal tract inflammation, weakened immune system, or decreased peristalsis; and
- injury to olfactory ensheathing glia can cause a loss of smell or a distorted sense of smell.

CST enhances PNS glia

Craniosacral therapy (CST) can reach PNS glia by transmitting corrective forces through the fascial matrix. Every cell and all structures are embedded within and interconnected by fascia. Fascia is a biomechanical connector and transmitter of forces. It is a web-like matrix of cells, proteins, molecules, and fluid that extends from every minuscule part of the body to adhere to the skin.

The skin can express underlying fascial patterns because the entire fascial matrix is one interconnected system. It is through this system that a CST practitioner can feel fascial patterns within another person's body. It is also through this system that corrective forces can be transmitted. Transmitting CST technique can help to correct many conditions in which PNS glia are involved, such as those listed above in the bullets.

In the following paragraphs, I will use DRG satellite glial cell disturbance as an example of how PNS glia can cause chronic pain. Then, I will show how that dysfunction can be corrected through CST techniques.

A DRG's environment can become overly stressed due to many causes, such as trauma, infection, spinal column misalignment, intervertebral disc dysfunction, spinal cord meningeal restriction, scar tissue, or nerve root compression. Even after a cause has been resolved, a ganglion can continue to be overly stressed, and this can lead to dysfunction, such as chronic pain.

Many conditions, such as those listed in the paragraph above, cause a sensation of pain. Sensory nerves transmitting pain signals can become overworked. Sensory nerve cell bodies are situated within dorsal root ganglia and are encased within satellite glia.

One important satellite glial cell job is to clear substances from the space immediately surrounding nerve cell bodies. When satellite glia are unable to perform this job quickly and efficiently, some of these substances can irritate nerve cell bodies, cause neuronal hyperexcitability, and bombard the spinal cord with excessive pain signals.

In response, hyperexcitability of spinal cord neurons takes place. Astrogliosis and microgliosis also occur, and this further elevates hyperexcitability. Spinal cord neuronal hyperexcitability is a cause of chronic pain.

CST techniques can reach dorsal root ganglion stress through the fascial matrix. Fascial components within a ganglion are interconnected to its surrounding fascia. The ganglion's surrounding fascia is interconnected to the entire fascial web. Inner ganglion stress can alter the outer shape of the ganglion. Since ganglion shape is coupled to the fascial web, its shape deformation is expressed throughout the entire fascial matrix, all the way to the skin.

Corrective forces can be transmitted through the same interconnected pathway into a dysfunctional ganglion or into a spinal cord area. These corrective forces can help soothe irritated nerves and glia, lessen inflammation, cleanse irritants, and thus lead to a resolution of chronic pain.

Infinite possibilities

CST techniques not only can reach into the depths of the body though the fascial system, they can also reach into the brain and spinal cord through the pia-glial interface (PGI) because the PGI interconnects fascia with the CNS glial cell matrix (glial syncytium).

Through the all-encompassing fascial-glial network, a practitioner can hold every cell in a person's body: from the deepest area of the brain to the surface of the skin. We have limitless possibilities of helping others overcome dysfunction. During each moment of CST, when we touch someone with a helping intention, we facilitate that person's boundless ability to heal. We are indeed fortunate to meet glia, "brain-star cells," through our hands. As we support glia, the stars of healing, we have the honor of entering a universe that transforms illness into health, dysfunction into vibrant life.

Bibliography

Abbott, N. J., and New York Academy of Sciences. 1991. Glial-neuronal interaction (Annals of the New York Academy of Sciences). New York: New York Academy of Sciences.

Abdo, H., P. Derkinderen, P. Gomes, J. Chevalier, P. Aubert, D. Masson, J. P. Galmiche, P. Vanden Berghe, M. Neunlist, and B. Lardeux. 2010. "Enteric glial cells protect neurons from oxidative stress in part via reduced glutathione." FASEB J 24 (4):1082-94. doi: 10.1096/fj.09-139519.

Agnati, L. F., S. Genedani, G. Leo, A. Rivera, D. Guidolin, and K. Fuxe. 2007. "One century of progress in neuroscience founded on Golgi and Cajal's outstanding experimental and theoretical contributions." Brain Res Rev 55 (1):167-89. doi: 10.1016/j.brainresrev.2007.03.004.

Agnati, L. F., D. Guidolin, M. Guescini, S. Genedani, and K. Fuxe. 2010. "Understanding wiring and volume transmission." Brain Res Rev 64 (1):137-59. doi: 10.1016/j.brainresrev.2010.03.003.

Agte, S., S. Junek, S. Matthias, E. Ulbricht, I. Erdmann, A. Wurm, D. Schild, J. A. Kas, and A. Reichenbach. 2011. "Muller glial cell-provided cellular light guidance through the vital guinea-pig retina." Biophys J 101 (11):2611-9. doi: 10.1016/j.bpj.2011.09.062.

Agulhon, C., M. Y. Sun, T. Murphy, T. Myers, K. Lauderdale, and T. A. Fiacco. 2012. "Calcium Signaling and Gliotransmission in Normal vs. Reactive Astrocytes." Front Pharmacol 3:139. doi: 10.3389/fphar.2012.00139.

Aguzzi, A., B. A. Barres, and M. L. Bennett. 2013. "Microglia: scapegoat, saboteur, or something else?" Science 339 (6116):156-61. doi: 10.1126/science.1227901.

Al Ahmad, A., M. Gassmann, and O. O. Ogunshola. 2009. "Maintaining blood-brain barrier integrity: pericytes perform better than astrocytes during prolonged oxygen deprivation." J Cell Physiol 218 (3):612-22. doi: 10.1002/jcp.21638.

Al Ahmad, A., C. B. Taboada, M. Gassmann, and O. O. Ogunshola. 2011. "Astrocytes and pericytes differentially modulate blood-brain barrier characteristics during development and hypoxic insult." J Cereb Blood Flow Metab 31 (2):693-705. doi: 10.1038/jcbfm.2010.148.

Allan, Frank D. 1969. Essentials of human embryology. 2nd ed. New York: Oxford University Press.

Almad, A. A., and N. J. Maragakis. 2012. "Glia: an emerging target for neurological disease therapy." Stem Cell Res Ther 3 (5):37. doi: 10.1186/scrt128.

Alvarez-Leefmans, F. J., John M. Russell, and International Brain Research Organization. Congress. 1990. Chloride channels and carriers in nerve, muscle, and glial cells. New York: Plenum Press.

Amiry-Moghaddam, M., and O. P. Ottersen. 2003. "The molecular basis of water transport in the brain." Nat Rev Neurosci 4 (12):991-1001. doi: 10.1038/nrn1252.

Anastassiou, C. A., R. Perin, H. Markram, and C. Koch. 2011. "Ephaptic coupling of cortical neurons." Nat Neurosci 14 (2):217-23. doi: 10.1038/nn.2727.

Anderson, M. A., Y. Ao, and M. V. Sofroniew. 2014. "Heterogeneity of reactive astrocytes." Neurosci Lett 565:23-9. doi: 10.1016/j.neulet.2013.12.030.

Araque, A., and M. Navarrete. 2010. "Glial cells in neuronal network function." Philos Trans R Soc Lond B Biol Sci 365 (1551):2375-81. doi: 10.1098/rstb.2009.0313.

Araque, A., V. Parpura, R. P. Sanzgiri, and P. G. Haydon. 1999. "Tripartite synapses: glia, the unacknowledged partner." Trends Neurosci 22 (5):208-15.

Armulik, A., A. Abramsson, and C. Betsholtz. 2005. "Endothelial/pericyte interactions." Circ Res 97 (6):512-23. doi: 10.1161/01.RES.0000182903.16652.d7.

Attwell, D., A. M. Buchan, S. Charpak, M. Lauritzen, B. A. Macvicar, and E. A. Newman. 2010. "Glial and neuronal control of brain blood flow." Nature 468 (7321):232-43. doi: 10.1038/nature09613.

Barker, A. J., and E. M. Ullian. 2008. "New roles for astrocytes in developing synaptic circuits." Commun Integr Biol 1 (2):207-11.

Barres, B. A. 2008. "The mystery and magic of glia: a perspective on their roles in health and disease." Neuron 60 (3):430-40. doi: 10.1016/j.neuron.2008.10.013.

Barry, D. S., J. M. Pakan, and K. W. McDermott. 2014. "Radial glial cells: key organisers in CNS development." Int J Biochem Cell Biol 46:76-9. doi: 10.1016/j.biocel.2013.11.013.

Baumann, N., and D. Pham-Dinh. 2001. "Biology of oligodendrocyte and myelin in the mammalian central nervous system." Physiol Rev 81 (2):871-927.

Bell, R. D., E. A. Winkler, A. P. Sagare, I. Singh, B. LaRue, R. Deane, and B. V. Zlokovic. 2010. "Pericytes control key neurovascular functions and neuronal phenotype in the adult brain and during brain aging." Neuron 68 (3):409-27. doi: 10.1016/j.neuron.2010.09.043.

Bergers, G., and S. Song. 2005. "The role of pericytes in blood-vessel formation and maintenance." Neuro Oncol 7 (4):452-64. doi: 10.1215/S1152851705000232.

Betsholtz, C. 2014. "Physiology: Double function at the blood-brain barrier." Nature 509 (7501):432-3. doi: 10.1038/nature13339.

Bezanilla, F. 2008. "Ion channels: from conductance to structure." Neuron 60 (3):456-68. doi: 10.1016/j.neuron.2008.10.035.

Binder, D. K., M. C. Papadopoulos, P. M. Haggie, and A. S. Verkman. 2004. "In vivo measurement of brain extracellular space diffusion by cortical surface photobleaching." J Neurosci 24 (37):8049-56. doi: 10.1523/JNEUROSCI.2294-04.2004.

Bjorklund, A., and C. Svendsen. 1999. "Stem cells. Breaking the brain-blood barrier." Nature 397 (6720):569-70. doi: 10.1038/17495.

Boron, Walter F., and Emile L. Boulpaep. 2012. Medical physiology: a cellular and molecular approach. Updated 2nd ed. Philadelphia, PA: Saunders/Elsevier.

Borrell, V., and M. Gotz. 2014. "Role of radial glial cells in cerebral cortex folding." Curr Opin Neurobiol 27:39-46. doi: 10.1016/j.conb.2014.02.007.

Brazhe, A. R., N. A. Brazhe, N. N. Rodionova, A. I. Yusipovich, P. S. Ignatyev, G. V. Maksimov, E. Mosekilde, and O. V. Sosnovtseva. 2008. "Non-invasive study of nerve fibres using laser interference microscopy." Philos Trans A Math Phys Eng Sci 366 (1880):3463-81. doi: 10.1098/rsta.2008.0107.

Brodal, Per. 2004. The central nervous system: structure and function. 3rd ed. Oxford; New York: Oxford University Press.

Brown, G. C., and A. Bal-Price. 2003. "Inflammatory neurodegeneration mediated by nitric oxide, glutamate, and mitochondria." Mol Neurobiol 27 (3):325-55. doi: 10.1385/MN:27:3:325.

Brown, G. C., and J. J. Neher. 2010. "Inflammatory neurodegeneration and mechanisms of microglial killing of neurons." Mol Neurobiol 41 (2-3):242-7. doi: 10.1007/s12035-010-8105-9.

Brunne, B., S. Zhao, A. Derouiche, J. Herz, P. May, M. Frotscher, and H. H. Bock. 2010. "Origin, maturation, and astroglial transformation of secondary radial glial cells in the developing dentate gyrus." Glia 58 (13):1553-69. doi: 10.1002/glia.21029.

Burdett, T. C., and M. R. Freeman. 2014. "Neuroscience. Astrocytes eyeball axonal mitochondria." Science 345 (6195):385-6. doi: 10.1126/science.1258295.

Buskila, Y., Y. Abu-Ghanem, Y. Levi, A. Moran, E. Grauer, and Y. Amitai. 2007. "Enhanced astrocytic nitric oxide production and neuronal modifications in the neocortex of a NOS2 mutant mouse." PLoS One 2 (9):e843. doi: 10.1371/journal.pone.0000843.

Butt, A. M., M. Pugh, P. Hubbard, and G. James. 2004. "Functions of optic nerve glia: axoglial signalling in physiology and pathology." Eye (Lond) 18 (11):1110-21. doi: 10.1038/sj.eye.6701595.

Byrne, John H., and James Lewis Roberts. 2009. From molecules to networks: an introduction to cellular and molecular neuroscience. 2nd ed. Amsterdam; Boston: Academic Press/Elsevier.

Cameron, R. S., and P. Rakic. 1991. "Glial cell lineage in the cerebral cortex: a review and synthesis." Glia 4 (2):124-37. doi: 10.1002/glia.440040204.

Carlson, Bruce M., and Bruce M. Carlson. 2004. Human embryology and developmental biology. 3rd ed. St. Louis, MO: Mosby.

Carmignoto, G., and P. G. Haydon. 2012. "Astrocyte calcium signaling and epilepsy." Glia 60 (8):1227-33. doi: 10.1002/glia.22318.

Chen, M. J., B. Kress, X. Han, K. Moll, W. Peng, R. R. Ji, and M. Nedergaard. 2012. "Astrocytic CX43 hemichannels and gap junctions play a crucial role in development of chronic neuropathic pain following spinal cord injury." Glia 60 (11):1660-70. doi: 10.1002/glia.22384.

Chikly, B., and J. Quaghebeur. 2013. "Reassessing cerebrospinal fluid (CSF) hydrodynamics: a literature review presenting a novel hypothesis for CSF physiology." J Bodyw Mov Ther 17 (3):344-54. doi: 10.1016/j.jbmt.2013.02.002.

Clasadonte, J., J. Dong, D. J. Hines, and P. G. Haydon. 2013. "Astrocyte control of synaptic NMDA receptors contributes to the progressive development of temporal lobe epilepsy." Proc Natl Acad Sci U S A 110 (43):17540-5. doi: 10.1073/pnas.1311967110.

Cochard, Larry R., and Frank H. Netter. 2002. Netter's atlas of human embryology. 1st ed. Teterboro, NJ: Icon Learning Systems.

Coiret, G., J. Ster, B. Grewe, F. Wendling, F. Helmchen, U. Gerber, and P. Benquet. 2012. "Neuron to astrocyte communication via cannabinoid receptors is necessary for sustained epileptiform activity in rat hippocampus." PLoS One 7 (5):e37320. doi: 10.1371/journal.pone.0037320.

Corona, C., C. Porcario, F. Martucci, B. Iulini, B. Manea, M. Gallo, C. Palmitessa, C. Maurella, M. Mazza, M. Pezzolato, P. Acutis, and C. Casalone. 2009. "Olfactory system involvement in natural scrapie disease." J Virol 83 (8):3657-67. doi: 10.1128/JVI.01966-08.

Czeh, B., E. Fuchs, and G. Flugge. 2013. "Altered glial plasticity in animal models for mood disorders." Curr Drug Targets 14 (11):1249-61.

Damkier, H. H., P. D. Brown, and J. Praetorius. 2013. "Cerebrospinal fluid secretion by the choroid plexus." Physiol Rev 93 (4):1847-92. doi: 10.1152/physrev.00004.2013.

Decimo, I., G. Fumagalli, V. Berton, M. Krampera, and F. Bifari. 2012. "Meninges: from protective membrane to stem cell niche." Am J Stem Cells 1 (2):92-105.

DeFelipe, Javier, and Santiago Ramón y Cajal. 2010. Cajal's butterflies of the soul: science and art. Oxford; New York: Oxford University Press.

Dirnagl, Ulrich, and B. Elger. 2004. Neuroinflammation in stroke, Ernst Schering Research Foundation workshop. Berlin; New York: Springer.

Dityatev, A., and M. Schachner. 2003. "Extracellular matrix molecules and synaptic plasticity." Nat Rev Neurosci 4 (6):456-68. doi: 10.1038/nrn1115.

Dityatev, A., C. I. Seidenbecher, and M. Schachner. 2010. "Compartmentalization from the outside: the extracellular matrix and functional microdomains in the brain." Trends Neurosci 33 (11):503-12. doi: 10.1016/j.tins.2010.08.003.

Dublin, P., and M. Hanani. 2007. "Satellite glial cells in sensory ganglia: their possible contribution to inflammatory pain." Brain Behav Immun 21 (5):592-8. doi: 10.1016/j.bbi.2006.11.011.

Dudek, F. E., and M. A. Rogawski. 2005. "Regulation of brain water: is there a role for aquaporins in epilepsy?" Epilepsy Curr 5 (3):104-6. doi: 10.1111/j.1535-7511.2005.05310.x.

Egelman, D. M., and P. R. Montague. 1999. "Calcium dynamics in the extracellular space of mammalian neural tissue." Biophys J 76 (4):1856-67.

Elenkov, I. J., R. L. Wilder, G. P. Chrousos, and E. S. Vizi. 2000. "The sympathetic nerve--an integrative interface between two supersystems: the brain and the immune system." Pharmacol Rev 52 (4):595-638.

Ernst, C., C. Nagy, S. Kim, J. P. Yang, X. Deng, I. C. Hellstrom, K. H. Choi, H. Gershenfeld, M. J. Meaney, and G. Turecki. 2011. "Dysfunction of astrocyte connexins 30 and 43 in dorsal lateral prefrontal cortex of suicide completers." Biol Psychiatry 70 (4):312-9. doi: 10.1016/j.biopsych.2011.03.038.

Etchevers, H. C., G. Couly, C. Vincent, and N. M. Le Douarin. 1999. "Anterior cephalic neural crest is required for forebrain viability." Development 126 (16):3533-43.

Euston, D. R., and H. W. Steenland. 2014. "Neuroscience. Memories—getting wired during sleep." Science 344 (6188):1087-8. doi: 10.1126/science.1255649.

Fatemi, S. H., T. D. Folsom, T. J. Reutiman, and S. Lee. 2008. "Expression of astrocytic markers aquaporin 4 and connexin 43 is altered in brains of subjects with autism." Synapse 62 (7):501-7. doi: 10.1002/syn.20519.

Faulkner, J. R., J. E. Herrmann, M. J. Woo, K. E. Tansey, N. B. Doan, and M. V. Sofroniew. 2004. "Reactive astrocytes protect tissue and preserve function after spinal cord injury." J Neurosci 24 (9):2143-55. doi: 10.1523/JNEUROSCI.3547-03.2004.

Felten, David L., Anil Narsinha Shetty, and David L. Felten. 2010. Netter's atlas of neuroscience. 2nd ed. Philadelphia, PA: Saunders/Elsevier.

Fields, R. Douglas. 2008. Beyond the synapse: cell-cell signaling in synaptic plasticity. Cambridge, UK; New York: Cambridge University Press.

Fields, R. D. 2010. "Central role of glia in disease research." Neuron Glia Biol 6 (2):91-2. doi: 10.1017/S1740925X10000177.

Fields, R. D. 2014. "Myelin formation and remodeling." Cell 156 (1-2):15-7. doi: 10.1016/j.cell.2013.12.038.

Fields, R. D. 2014. "Neuroscience. Myelin—more than insulation." Science 344 (6181):264-6. doi: 10.1126/science.1253851.

Florence, C. M., L. D. Baillie, and S. J. Mulligan. 2012. "Dynamic volume changes in astrocytes are an intrinsic phenomenon mediated by bicarbonate ion flux." PLoS One 7 (11):e51124. doi: 10.1371/journal.pone.0051124.

Franze, K., J. Grosche, S. N. Skatchkov, S. Schinkinger, C. Foja, D. Schild, O. Uckermann, K. Travis, A. Reichenbach, and J. Guck. 2007. "Muller cells are living optical fibers in the vertebrate retina." Proc Natl Acad Sci U S A 104 (20):8287-92. doi: 10.1073/pnas.0611180104.

Fraser, J. R., T. C. Laurent, and U. B. Laurent. 1997. "Hyaluronan: its nature, distribution, functions and turnover." J Intern Med 242 (1):27-33.

Furness, John Barton. 2006. The enteric nervous system. Malden, MA: Blackwell Publishing.

Gaengel, K., G. Genove, A. Armulik, and C. Betsholtz. 2009. "Endothelial-mural cell signaling in vascular development and angiogenesis." Arterioscler Thromb Vasc Biol 29 (5):630-8. doi: 10.1161/ATVBAHA.107.161521.

Garcia, M., and E. Vecino. 2003. "Role of Muller glia in neuroprotection and regeneration in the retina." Histol Histopathol 18 (4):1205-18.

Gato, A., and M. E. Desmond. 2009. "Why the embryo still matters: CSF and the neuroepithelium as interdependent regulators of embryonic brain growth, morphogenesis and histiogenesis." Dev Biol 327 (2):263-72. doi: 10.1016/j.ydbio.2008.12.029.

Gaudet, A. D., P. G. Popovich, and M. S. Ramer. 2011. "Wallerian degeneration: gaining perspective on inflammatory events after peripheral nerve injury." J Neuroinflammation 8:110. doi: 10.1186/1742-2094-8-110.

Gire, D. H., K. M. Franks, J. D. Zak, K. F. Tanaka, J. D. Whitesell, A. A. Mulligan, R. Hen, and N. E. Schoppa. 2012. "Mitral cells in the olfactory bulb are mainly excited through a multistep signaling path." J Neurosci 32 (9):2964-75. doi: 10.1523/J Neurosci.5580-11.2012.

González Pérez, Oscar. 2012. Astrocytes: structure, functions and role in disease, Neuroscience research progress. New York: Nova Science Publishers.

Gotz, M., and W. B. Huttner. 2005. "The cell biology of neurogenesis." Nat Rev Mol Cell Biol 6 (10):777-88. doi: 10.1038/nrm1739.

Grathwohl, S. A., R. E. Kalin, T. Bolmont, S. Prokop, G. Winkelmann, S. A. Kaeser, J. Odenthal, R. Radde, T. Eldh, S. Gandy, A. Aguzzi, M. Staufenbiel, P. M. Mathews, H. Wolburg, F. L. Heppner, and M. Jucker. 2009. "Formation and maintenance of Alzheimer's disease beta-amyloid plaques in the absence of microglia." Nat Neurosci 12 (11):1361-3. doi: 10.1038/nn.2432.

Gray, Henry, Susan Standring, Harold Ellis, and B. K. B. Berkovitz. 2005. Gray's anatomy: the anatomical basis of clinical practice. 39th ed. Edinburgh; New York: Elsevier Churchill Livingstone.

Gregg, C. T., A. K. Chojnacki, and S. Weiss. 2002. "Radial glial cells as neuronal precursors: the next generation?" J Neurosci Res 69 (6):708-13. doi: 10.1002/jnr.10340.

Guillery, R. W. 2005. "Observations of synaptic structures: origins of the neuron doctrine and its current status." Philos Trans R Soc Lond B Biol Sci 360 (1458):1281-307. doi: 10.1098/rstb.2003.1459.

Gupta, S., M. Soellinger, D. M. Grzybowski, P. Boesiger, J. Biddiscombe, D. Poulikakos, and V. Kurtcuoglu. 2010. "Cerebrospinal fluid dynamics in the human cranial subarachnoid space: an overlooked mediator of cerebral disease. I. Computational model." J R Soc Interface 7 (49):1195-204. doi: 10.1098/rsif.2010.0033.

Hall, A. P. 2006. "Review of the pericyte during angiogenesis and its role in cancer and diabetic retinopathy." Toxicol Pathol 34 (6):763-75. doi: 10.1080/01926230600936290.

Hall, John E., and Arthur C. Guyton. 2011. Guyton and Hall textbook of medical physiology. 12th ed. Philadelphia, PA: Saunders/Elsevier.

Hamby, M. E., and M. V. Sofroniew. 2010. "Reactive astrocytes as therapeutic targets for CNS disorders." Neurotherapeutics 7 (4):494-506. doi: 10.1016/j.nurt.2010.07.003.

Hanani, M. 2005. "Satellite glial cells in sensory ganglia: from form to function." Brain Res Brain Res Rev 48 (3):457-76. doi: 10.1016/j.brainresrev.2004.09.001.

Hansen, D. V., J. H. Lui, P. R. Parker, and A. R. Kriegstein. 2010. "Neurogenic radial glia in the outer subventricular zone of human neocortex." Nature 464 (7288):554-561. doi: 10.1038/nature08845.

Hansson, E. 2006. "Could chronic pain and spread of pain sensation be induced and maintained by glial activation?" Acta Physiol (Oxf) 187 (1-2):321-7. doi: 10.1111/j.1748-1716.2006.01568.x.

Hansson, E., and L. Ronnback. 2003. "Glial neuronal signaling in the central nervous system." FASEB J 17 (3):341-8. doi: 10.1096/fj.02-0429rev.

Hansson, E., and R. Zugner. 2005. "Can chronic pain and spreading of pain be induced via glial mechanisms? New hypotheses on the generators maintaining protracted pain conditions." Lakartidningen 102 (47):3552, 3555-6, 3558.

Hawkins, B. T., and T. P. Davis. 2005. "The blood-brain barrier/neurovascular unit in health and disease." Pharmacol Rev 57 (2):173-85. doi: 10.1124/pr.57.2.4.

Hayashi, Y., M. Nomura, S. Yamagishi, S. Harada, J. Yamashita, and H. Yamamoto. 1997. "Induction of various blood-brain barrier properties in non-neural endothelial cells by close apposition to co-cultured astrocytes." Glia 19 (1):13-26.

Haydon, P. G., and G. Carmignoto. 2006. "Astrocyte control of synaptic transmission and neurovascular coupling." Physiol Rev 86 (3):1009-31. doi: 10.1152/physrev.00049.2005.

Iliff, J. J., H. Lee, M. Yu, T. Feng, J. Logan, M. Nedergaard, and H. Benveniste. 2013. "Brain-wide pathway for waste clearance captured by contrast-enhanced MRI." J Clin Invest 123 (3):1299-309. doi: 10.1172/JCI67677.

Iliff, J. J., M. Wang, Y. Liao, B. A. Plogg, W. Peng, G. A. Gundersen, H. Benveniste, G. E. Vates, R. Deane, S. A. Goldman, E. A. Nagelhus, and M. Nedergaard. 2012. "A paravascular pathway facilitates CSF flow through the brain parenchyma and the clearance of interstitial solutes, including amyloid beta." Sci Transl Med 4 (147):147ra111. doi: 10.1126/scitranslmed.3003748.

Ingber, D. E. 2008. "Tensegrity and mechanotransduction." J Bodyw Mov Ther 12 (3):198-200. doi: 10.1016/j.jbmt.2008.04.038.

Inglese, M., E. Bomsztyk, O. Gonen, L. J. Mannon, R. I. Grossman, and H. Rusinek. 2005. "Dilated perivascular spaces: hallmarks of mild traumatic brain injury." AJNR Am J Neuroradiol 26 (4):719-24.

Isasi, E., L. Barbeito, and S. Olivera-Bravo. 2014. "Increased blood-brain barrier permeability and alterations in perivascular astrocytes and pericytes induced by intracisternal glutaric acid." Fluids Barriers CNS 11:15. doi: 10.1186/2045-8118-11-15.

Jasmin, L., J. P. Vit, A. Bhargava, and P. T. Ohara. 2010. "Can satellite glial cells be therapeutic targets for pain control?" Neuron Glia Biol 6 (1):63-71. doi: 10.1017/S1740925X10000098.

Jessen, K. R. 2004. "Glial cells." Int J Biochem Cell Biol 36 (10):1861-7. doi: 10.1016/j.biocel.2004.02.023.

Jessen, K. R., and R. Mirsky. 2005. "The origin and development of glial cells in peripheral nerves." Nat Rev Neurosci 6 (9):671-82. doi: 10.1038/nrn1746.

Ji, R. R., T. Berta, and M. Nedergaard. 2013. "Glia and pain: is chronic pain a gliopathy?" Pain 154 Suppl 1:S10-28. doi: 10.1016/j.pain.2013.06.022.

Johanson, C., E. Stopa, P. McMillan, D. Roth, J. Funk, and G. Krinke. 2011. "The distributional nexus of choroid plexus to cerebrospinal fluid, ependyma and brain: toxicologic/pathologic phenomena, periventricular destabilization, and lesion spread." Toxicol Pathol 39 (1):186-212. doi: 10.1177/0192623310394214.

Johanson, C. E., J. A. Duncan, 3rd, P. M. Klinge, T. Brinker, E. G. Stopa, and G. D. Silverberg. 2008. "Multiplicity of cerebrospinal fluid functions: New challenges in health and disease." Cerebrospinal Fluid Res 5:10. doi: 10.1186/1743-8454-5-10.

Jourdain, P., L. H. Bergersen, K. Bhaukaurally, P. Bezzi, M. Santello, M. Domercq, C. Matute, F. Tonello, V. Gundersen, and A. Volterra. 2007. "Glutamate exocytosis from astrocytes controls synaptic strength." Nat Neurosci 10 (3):331-9. doi: 10.1038/nn1849.

Kettenmann, Helmut, Helmut Kettenmann, and Bruce R. Ransom. 2013. Neuroglia. 3rd ed. Oxford; New York: Oxford University Press.

Kevany, B. M., and K. Palczewski. 2010. "Phagocytosis of retinal rod and cone photoreceptors." Physiology (Bethesda) 25 (1):8-15. doi: 10.1152/physiol.00038.2009.

Khakh, B. S., and M. V. Sofroniew. 2014. "Astrocytes and Huntington's disease." ACS Chem Neurosci 5 (7):494-6. doi: 10.1021/cn500100r.

Killer, H. E., G. P. Jaggi, J. Flammer, N. R. Miller, and A. R. Huber. 2006. "The optic nerve: a new window into cerebrospinal fluid composition?" Brain 129 (Pt 4):1027-30. doi: 10.1093/brain/awl045.

Killer, H. E., H. R. Laeng, J. Flammer, and P. Groscurth. 2003. "Architecture of arachnoid trabeculae, pillars, and septa in the subarachnoid space of the human optic nerve: anatomy and clinical considerations." Br J Ophthalmol 87 (6):777-81.

Kim, D. S., P. J. Ross, K. Zaslavsky, and J. Ellis. 2014. "Optimizing neuronal differentiation from induced pluripotent stem cells to model ASD." Front Cell Neurosci 8:109. doi: 10.3389/fncel.2014.00109.

Kim, H. J., and W. Sun. 2012. "Adult neurogenesis in the central and peripheral nervous systems." Int Neurourol J 16 (2):57-61. doi: 10.5213/inj.2012.16.2.57.

Klarica, M., B. Mise, A. Vladic, M. Rados, and D. Oreskovic. 2013. "Compensated hyperosmolarity of cerebrospinal fluid and the development of hydrocephalus." Neuroscience 248C:278-289. doi: 10.1016/j.neuroscience.2013.06.022.

Klarica, M., and D. Oreskovic. 2014. "Enigma of cerebrospinal fluid dynamics." Croat Med J 55 (4):287-90.

Koh, L., A. Zakharov, and M. Johnston. 2005. "Integration of the subarachnoid space and lymphatics: is it time to embrace a new concept of cerebrospinal fluid absorption?" Cerebrospinal Fluid Res 2:6. doi: 10.1186/1743-8454-2-6.

Koob, Andrew. 2009. The root of thought: unlocking glia—the brain cell that will help us sharpen our wits, heal injury, and treat brain disease. Upper Saddle River, NJ: FT Press.

Krzyzanowska, A., and E. Carro. 2012. "Pathological alteration in the choroid plexus of Alzheimer's disease: implication for new therapy approaches." Front Pharmacol 3:75. doi: 10.3389/fphar.2012.00075.

Kuchler-Bopp, S., J. P. Delaunoy, J. C. Artault, M. Zaepfel, and J. B. Dietrich. 1999. "Astrocytes induce several blood-brain barrier properties in non-neural endothelial cells." Neuroreport 10 (6):1347-53.

Kuo, Y. C., and C. H. Lu. 2011. "Effect of human astrocytes on the characteristics of human brain-microvascular endothelial cells in the blood-brain barrier." Colloids Surf B Biointerfaces 86 (1):225-31. doi: 10.1016/j.colsurfb.2011.04.005.

Larsen, William J. 1998. Essentials of human embryology. New York: Churchill Livingstone.

LeBleu, V. S., B. Macdonald, and R. Kalluri. 2007. "Structure and function of basement membranes." Exp Biol Med (Maywood) 232 (9):1121-9. doi: 10.3181/0703-MR-72.

Lee, H. S., A. Ghetti, A. Pinto-Duarte, X. Wang, G. Dziewczapolski, F. Galimi, S. Huitron-Resendiz, J. C. Pina-Crespo, A. J. Roberts, I. M. Verma, T. J. Sejnowski, and S. F. Heinemann. 2014. "Astrocytes contribute to gamma oscillations and recognition memory." Proc Natl Acad Sci U S A 111 (32):E3343-52. doi: 10.1073/pnas.1410893111.

Lehmann, G. L., S. A. Gradilone, and R. A. Marinelli. 2004. "Aquaporin water channels in central nervous system." Curr Neurovasc Res 1 (4):293-303.

Levison, Steven W. 2006. Mammalian subventricular zones: their roles in brain development, cell replacement, and disease. New York: Springer.

Li, T., J. Q. Lan, and D. Boison. 2008. "Uncoupling of astrogliosis from epileptogenesis in adenosine kinase (ADK) transgenic mice." Neuron Glia Biol 4 (2):91-9. doi: 10.1017/S1740925X09990135.

Liem, Torsten. 2004. Cranial osteopathy: principles and practice. 2nd ed. Edinburgh; New York: Elsevier Churchill Livingstone.

Lindsay, Mark, and Chad Robertson. 2008. Fascia: clinical applications for health and human performance. Clifton Park, NY: Delmar.

Lindvall, M., and C. Owman. 1981. "Autonomic nerves in the mammalian choroid plexus and their influence on the formation of cerebrospinal fluid." J Cereb Blood Flow Metab 1 (3):245-66. doi: 10.1038/jcbfm.1981.30.

Loov, C., L. Hillered, T. Ebendal, and A. Erlandsson. 2012. "Engulfing astrocytes protect neurons from contact-induced apoptosis following injury." PLoS One 7 (3):e33090. doi: 10.1371/journal.pone.0033090.

Losi, G., M. Cammarota, and G. Carmignoto. 2012. "The role of astroglia in the epileptic brain." Front Pharmacol 3:132. doi: 10.3389/fphar.2012.00132.

Lubischer, J. L., and D. M. Bebinger. 1999. "Regulation of terminal Schwann cell number at the adult neuromuscular junction." J Neurosci 19 (24):RC46.

Mack, A. F., and H. Wolburg. 2013. "A novel look at astrocytes: aquaporins, ionic homeostasis, and the role of the microenvironment for regeneration in the CNS." Neuroscientist 19 (2):195-207. doi: 10.1177/1073858412447981.

Marin, O. 2012. "Brain development: The neuron family tree remodelled." Nature 490 (7419):185-6. doi: 10.1038/490185a.

McCoy, E., and H. Sontheimer. 2007. "Expression and function of water channels (aquaporins) in migrating malignant astrocytes." Glia 55 (10):1034-43. doi: 10.1002/glia.20524.

Miller, Karol. 2011. "Biomechanics of the brain." In Biological and medical physics, biomedical engineering. New York: Springer.

Miranda, R. C. 2012. "MicroRNAs and fetal brain development: implications for ethanol teratology during the second trimester period of neurogenesis." Front Genet 3:77. doi: 10.3389/fgene.2012.00077.

Mithal, D. S., D. Ren, and R. J. Miller. 2013. "CXCR4 signaling regulates radial glial morphology and cell fate during embryonic spinal cord development." Glia 61 (8):1288-305. doi: 10.1002/glia.22515.

Moore, Keith L., T. V. N. Persaud, and Mark G. Torchia. 2013. Before we are born: essentials of embryology and birth defects. 8th ed. Philadelphia, PA: Saunders/Elsevier.

Mori, S., S. Wakana, and P. C. M. Van Zijl. 2004. MRI atlas of human white matter. 1st ed. Amsterdam; San Diego, CA: Elsevier.

Morris, A. W., R. O. Carare, S. Schreiber, and C. A. Hawkes. 2014. "The cerebrovascular basement membrane: role in the clearance of beta-amyloid and cerebral amyloid angiopathy." Front Aging Neurosci 6:251. doi: 10.3389/fnagi.2014.00251.

Mustafa, A. K., P. M. Kim, and S. H. Snyder. 2004. "D-Serine as a putative glial neurotransmitter." Neuron Glia Biol 1 (3):275-81. doi: 10.1017/S1740925X05000141.

Myer, D. J., G. G. Gurkoff, S. M. Lee, D. A. Hovda, and M. V. Sofroniew. 2006. "Essential protective roles of reactive astrocytes in traumatic brain injury." Brain 129 (Pt 10):2761-72. doi: 10.1093/brain/awl165.

Nagra, G., L. Koh, A. Zakharov, D. Armstrong, and M. Johnston. 2006. "Quantification of cerebrospinal fluid transport across the cribriform plate into lymphatics in rats." Am J Physiol Regul Integr Comp Physiol 291 (5):R1383-9. doi: 10.1152/ajpregu.00235.2006.

Nagy, J. I., A. V. Ionescu, B. D. Lynn, and J. E. Rash. 2003. "Coupling of astrocyte connexins Cx26, Cx30, Cx43 to oligodendrocyte Cx29, Cx32, Cx47: Implications from normal and connexin32 knockout mice." Glia 44 (3):205-18. doi: 10.1002/glia.10278.

Nagy, J. I., and J. E. Rash. 2003. "Astrocyte and oligodendrocyte connexins of the glial syncytium in relation to astrocyte anatomical domains and spatial buffering." Cell Commun Adhes 10 (4-6):401-6.

Netter, Frank H. 2014. Atlas of human anatomy. 6th edition. ed. Philadelphia, PA: Saunders/Elsevier.

Newman, E., and A. Reichenbach. 1996. "The Muller cell: a functional element of the retina." Trends Neurosci 19 (8):307-12.

Newman, L. A., D. L. Korol, and P. E. Gold. 2011. "Lactate produced by glycogenolysis in astrocytes regulates memory processing." PLoS One 6 (12):e28427. doi: 10.1371/journal.pone.0028427.

Ohara, P. T., J. P. Vit, A. Bhargava, M. Romero, C. Sundberg, A. C. Charles, and L. Jasmin. 2009. "Gliopathic pain: when satellite glial cells go bad." Neuroscientist 15 (5):450-63. doi: 10.1177/1073858409336094.

Ongur, D., A. J. Bechtholt, W. A. Carlezon, Jr., and B. M. Cohen. 2014. "Glial abnormalities in mood disorders." Harv Rev Psychiatry 22 (6):334-7. doi: 10.1097/HRP.60.

Oreskovic, D., and M. Klarica. 2010. "The formation of cerebrospinal fluid: nearly a hundred years of interpretations and misinterpretations." Brain Res Rev 64 (2):241-62. doi: 10.1016/j.brainresrev.2010.04.006.

Pajevic, S., P. J. Basser, and R. D. Fields. 2014. "Role of myelin plasticity in oscillations and synchrony of neuronal activity." Neuroscience 276:135-47. doi: 10.1016/j.neuroscience.2013.11.007.

Pannese, Ennio. 1994. Neurocytology: fine structure of neurons, nerve processes, and neuroglial cells. Stuttgart; New York: G. Thieme Verlag.

Paoletti, Serge. 2006. The fasciae: anatomy, dysfunction and treatment. English ed. Seattle: Eastland Press.

Papadopoulos, M. C., and A. S. Verkman. 2013. "Aquaporin water channels in the nervous system." Nat Rev Neurosci 14 (4):265-77. doi: 10.1038/nrn3468.

Park, J. B., H. J. Kwak, and S. H. Lee. 2008. "Role of hyaluronan in glioma invasion." Cell Adh Migr 2 (3):202-7.

Parpura, Vladimir, and Philip G. Haydon. 2009. Astrocytes in (patho)physiology of the nervous system. New York: Springer.

Perea, G., M. Navarrete, and A. Araque. 2009. "Tripartite synapses: astrocytes process and control synaptic information." Trends Neurosci 32 (8):421-31. doi: 10.1016/j.tins.2009.05.001.

Perez-Alvarez, A., and A. Araque. 2013. "Astrocyte-neuron interaction at tripartite synapses." Curr Drug Targets 14 (11):1220-4.

Perrin, R. N. 2007. "Lymphatic drainage of the neuraxis in chronic fatigue syndrome: a hypothetical model for the cranial rhythmic impulse." J Am Osteopath Assoc 107 (6):218-24.

Peterson, E. C., Z. Wang, and G. Britz. 2011. "Regulation of cerebral blood flow." Int J Vasc Med 2011:823525. doi: 10.1155/2011/823525.

Petzold, G. C., and V. N. Murthy. 2011. "Role of astrocytes in neurovascular coupling." Neuron 71 (5):782-97. doi: 10.1016/j.neuron.2011.08.009.

Pischinger, Alfred, and Hartmut Heine. 2007. The extracellular matrix and ground regulation: basis for a holistic biological medicine. Berkeley, CA: North Atlantic Books.

Pollay, M. 2010. "The function and structure of the cerebrospinal fluid outflow system." Cerebrospinal Fluid Res 7:9. doi: 10.1186/1743-8454-7-9.

Polyak, Stephen Lucian. 1941. The retina; the anatomy and the histology of the retina in man, ape, and monkey, including the consideration of visual functions, the history of physiological optics, and the histological laboratory technique. Chicago: The University of Chicago Press.

Preston, J. E. 2001. "Ageing choroid plexus-cerebrospinal fluid system." Microsc Res Tech 52 (1):31-7. doi: 10.1002/1097-0029(20010101)52:1<31::AID-JEMT5>3.0.CO;2-T.

Prevost, T. P., A. Balakrishnan, S. Suresh, and S. Socrate. 2011. "Biomechanics of brain tissue." Acta Biomater 7 (1):83-95. doi: 10.1016/j.actbio.2010.06.035.

Priller, J., M. Prinz, M. Heikenwalder, N. Zeller, P. Schwarz, F. L. Heppner, and A. Aguzzi. 2006. "Early and rapid engraftment of bone marrow-derived microglia in scrapie." J Neurosci 26 (45):11753-62. doi: 10.1523/JNEUROSCI.2275-06.2006.

Purves, Dale, and S. Mark Williams. 2001. Neuroscience. 2nd ed. Sunderland, MA: Sinauer Associates.

Redzic, Z. B., J. E. Preston, J. A. Duncan, A. Chodobski, and J. Szmydynger-Chodobska. 2005. "The choroid plexus-cerebrospinal fluid system: from development to aging." Curr Top Dev Biol 71:1-52. doi: 10.1016/S0070-2153(05)71001-2.

Riquelme, P. A., E. Drapeau, and F. Doetsch. 2008. "Brain micro-ecologies: neural stem cell niches in the adult mammalian brain." Philos Trans R Soc Lond B Biol Sci 363 (1489):123-37. doi: 10.1098/rstb.2006.2016.

Rogawski, M. A. 2005. "Astrocytes get in the act in epilepsy." Nat Med 11 (9):919-20. doi: 10.1038/nm0905-919.

Roth, T. L., D. Nayak, T. Atanasijevic, A. P. Koretsky, L. L. Latour, and D. B. McGavern. 2014. "Transcranial amelioration of inflammation and cell death after brain injury." Nature 505 (7482):223-8. doi: 10.1038/nature12808.

Rowitch, D. H., and A. R. Kriegstein. 2010. "Developmental genetics of vertebrate glial-cell specification." Nature 468 (7321):214-22. doi: 10.1038/nature09611.

Ruoslahti, E. 1996. "Brain extracellular matrix." Glycobiology 6 (5):489-92.

Sakka, L., G. Coll, and J. Chazal. 2011. "Anatomy and physiology of cerebrospinal fluid." Eur Ann Otorhinolaryngol Head Neck Dis 128 (6):309-16. doi: 10.1016/j.anorl.2011.03.002.

Sanai, N., T. Nguyen, R. A. Ihrie, Z. Mirzadeh, H. H. Tsai, M. Wong, N. Gupta, M. S. Berger, E. Huang, J. M. Garcia-Verdugo, D. H. Rowitch, and A. Alvarez-Buylla. 2011. "Corridors of migrating neurons in the human brain and their decline during infancy." Nature 478 (7369):382-6. doi: 10.1038/nature10487.

Sathyanesan, M., M. J. Girgenti, M. Banasr, K. Stone, C. Bruce, E. Guilchicek, K. Wilczak-Havill, A. Nairn, K. Williams, S. Sass, J. G. Duman, and S. S. Newton. 2012. "A molecular characterization of the choroid plexus and stress-induced gene regulation." Transl Psychiatry 2:e139. doi: 10.1038/tp.2012.64.

Scemes, Eliana, and David C. Spray. 2012. Astrocytes: wiring the brain, Frontiers in neuroscience. Boca Raton, FL: CRC Press.

Schipper, Hyman M. 1998. Astrocytes in brain aging and neurodegeneration, Neuroscience intelligence unit. Austin, TX: R.G. Landes.

Schleip, Robert. 2012. Fascia: the tensional network of the human body: the science and clinical applications in manual and movement therapy. Edinburgh; New York: Churchill Livingstone/Elsevier.

Schoenwolf, Gary C., Steven B. Bleyl, Philip R. Brauer, and P. H. Francis-West. 2015. Larsen's human embryology. 5th edition. Philadelphia, PA: Elsevier/Churchill Livingstone.

Schroeter, M. L., H. Abdul-Khaliq, J. Sacher, J. Steiner, I. E. Blasig, and K. Mueller. 2010. "Mood disorders are glial disorders: evidence from in vivo studies." Cardiovasc Psychiatry Neurol 2010:780645. doi: 10.1155/2010/780645.

Schwartz, M., and Y. Ziv. 2008. "Immunity to self and self-maintenance: a unified theory of brain pathologies." Trends Immunol 29 (5):211-9. doi: 10.1016/j.it.2008.01.003.

Skipor, J., and J. C. Thiery. 2008. "The choroid plexus—cerebrospinal fluid system: undervalued pathway of neuroendocrine signaling into the brain." Acta Neurobiol Exp (Wars) 68 (3):414-28.

Sofroniew, M. V. 2005. "Reactive astrocytes in neural repair and protection." Neuroscientist 11 (5):400-7. doi: 10.1177/1073858405278321.

Sofroniew, M. V. 2014. "Multiple roles for astrocytes as effectors of cytokines and inflammatory mediators." Neuroscientist 20 (2):160-72. doi: 10.1177/1073858413504466.

Sofroniew, M. V., and H. V. Vinters. 2010. "Astrocytes: biology and pathology." Acta Neuropathol 119 (1):7-35. doi: 10.1007/s00401-009-0619-8.

Sokolowski, J. D., and J. W. Mandell. 2011. "Phagocytic clearance in neurodegeneration." Am J Pathol 178 (4):1416-28. doi: 10.1016/j.ajpath.2010.12.051.

Squire, Larry R. 2013. Fundamental neuroscience. 4th ed. Amsterdam; Boston: Elsevier/Academic Press.

Strange, K. 1992. "Regulation of solute and water balance and cell volume in the central nervous system." J Am Soc Nephrol 3 (1):12-27.

Strittmatter, W. J. 2013. "Bathing the brain." J Clin Invest 123 (3):1013-5. doi: 10.1172/JCI68241.

Struckhoff, G. 1995. "Cocultures of meningeal and astrocytic cells--a model for the formation of the glial-limiting membrane." Int J Dev Neurosci 13 (6):595-606.

Sykova, E., and A. Chvatal. 2000. "Glial cells and volume transmission in the CNS." Neurochem Int 36 (4-5):397-409.

Takahashi, Y., D. Sipp, and H. Enomoto. 2013. "Tissue interactions in neural crest cell development and disease." Science 341 (6148):860-3. doi: 10.1126/science.1230717.

Tan, S. S. 2002. "Developmental neurobiology: cortical liars." Nature 417 (6889):605-6. doi: 10.1038/417605a.

Taverna, E., M. Gotz, and W. B. Huttner. 2014. "The Cell Biology of Neurogenesis: Toward an Understanding of the Development and Evolution of the Neocortex." Annu Rev Cell Dev Biol. doi: 10.1146/annurev-cellbio-101011-155801.

Temburni, M. K., and M. H. Jacob. 2001. "New functions for glia in the brain." Proc Natl Acad Sci U S A 98 (7):3631-2. doi: 10.1073/pnas.081073198.

Tramontin, A. D., J. M. Garcia-Verdugo, D. A. Lim, and A. Alvarez-Buylla. 2003. "Postnatal development of radial glia and the ventricular zone (VZ): a continuum of the neural stem cell compartment." Cereb Cortex 13 (6):580-7.

Turvey, M. T., and S. T. Fonseca. 2014. "The medium of haptic perception: a tensegrity hypothesis." J Mot Behav 46 (3):143-87. doi: 10.1080/00222895.2013.798252.

Upledger, John E., and Jon D. Vredevoogd. 1983. Craniosacral therapy. Chicago: Eastland Press.

Vargova, L., A. Chvatal, M. Anderova, S. Kubinova, D. Ziak, and E. Sykova. 2001. "Effect of osmotic stress on potassium accumulation around glial cells and extracellular space volume in rat spinal cord slices." J Neurosci Res 65 (2):129-38.

Vargova, L., and E. Sykova. 2014. "Astrocytes and extracellular matrix in extrasynaptic volume transmission." Philos Trans R Soc Lond B Biol Sci 369 (1654):20130608. doi: 10.1098/rstb.2013.0608.

Veening, J. G., and H. P. Barendregt. 2010. "The regulation of brain states by neuroactive substances distributed via the cerebrospinal fluid; a review." Cerebrospinal Fluid Res 7:1. doi: 10.1186/1743-8454-7-1.

Verkhratskii, A. N., and Arthur Butt. 2007. Glial neurobiology: a textbook. Chichester, UK; Hoboken, NJ: John Wiley & Sons.

Verkhratskii, A. N., and Arthur Butt. 2012. Glial physiology and pathophysiology: a handbook. Chichester, UK: John Wiley & Sons.

Verkhratsky, A. 2006. "Glial calcium signaling in physiology and pathophysiology." Acta Pharmacol Sin 27 (7):773-80. doi: 10.1111/j.1745-7254.2006.00396.x.

Vladic, A., M. Klarica, and M. Bulat. 2009. "Dynamics of distribution of 3H-inulin between the cerebrospinal fluid compartments." Brain Res 1248:127-35. doi: 10.1016/j.brainres.2008.10.044.

Voskuhl, R. R., R. S. Peterson, B. Song, Y. Ao, L. B. Morales, S. Tiwari-Woodruff, and M. V. Sofroniew. 2009. "Reactive astrocytes form scar-like perivascular barriers to leukocytes during adaptive immune inflammation of the CNS." J Neurosci 29 (37):11511-22. doi: 10.1523/JNEUROSCI.1514-09.2009.

Wang, J. T., Z. A. Medress, and B. A. Barres. 2012. "Axon degeneration: molecular mechanisms of a self-destruction pathway." J Cell Biol 196 (1):7-18. doi: 10.1083/jcb.201108111.

Wang, Q., D. A. Pelligrino, V. L. Baughman, H. M. Koenig, and R. F. Albrecht. 1995. "The role of neuronal nitric oxide synthase in regulation of cerebral blood flow in normocapnia and hypercapnia in rats." J Cereb Blood Flow Metab 15 (5):774-8. doi: 10.1038/jcbfm.1995.98.

Wanner, I. B., M. A. Anderson, B. Song, J. Levine, A. Fernandez, Z. Gray-Thompson, Y. Ao, and M. V. Sofroniew. 2013. "Glial scar borders are formed by newly proliferated, elongated astrocytes that interact to corral inflammatory and fibrotic cells via STAT3-dependent mechanisms after spinal cord injury." J Neurosci 33 (31):12870-86. doi: 10.1523/JNEUROSCI.2121-13.2013.

Whedon, J. M., and D. Glassey. 2009. "Cerebrospinal fluid stasis and its clinical significance." Altern Ther Health Med 15 (3):54-60.

Wiese, S., M. Karus, and A. Faissner. 2012. "Astrocytes as a source for extracellular matrix molecules and cytokines." Front Pharmacol 3:120. doi: 10.3389/fphar.2012.00120.

Wlodarczyk, J., I. Mukhina, L. Kaczmarek, and A. Dityatev. 2011. "Extracellular matrix molecules, their receptors, and secreted proteases in synaptic plasticity." Dev Neurobiol 71 (11):1040-53. doi: 10.1002/dneu.20958.

Xie, L., H. Kang, Q. Xu, M. J. Chen, Y. Liao, M. Thiyagarajan, J. O'Donnell, D. J. Christensen, C. Nicholson, J. J. Iliff, T. Takano, R. Deane, and M. Nedergaard. 2013. "Sleep drives metabolite clearance from the adult brain." Science 342 (6156):373-7. doi: 10.1126/science.1241224.

Yang, L., B. T. Kress, H. J. Weber, M. Thiyagarajan, B. Wang, R. Deane, H. Benveniste, J. J. Iliff, and M. Nedergaard. 2013. "Evaluating glymphatic pathway function utilizing clinically relevant intrathecal infusion of CSF tracer." J Transl Med 11:107. doi: 10.1186/1479-5876-11-107.

Yanguas-Casas, N., M. A. Barreda-Manso, M. Nieto-Sampedro, and L. Romero-Ramirez. 2014. "Tauroursodeoxycholic acid reduces glial cell activation in an animal model of acute neuroinflammation." J Neuroinflammation 11:50. doi: 10.1186/1742-2094-11-50.

Young, S. Z., M. M. Taylor, and A. Bordey. 2011. "Neurotransmitters couple brain activity to subventricular zone neurogenesis." Eur J Neurosci 33 (6):1123-32. doi: 10.1111/j.1460-9568.2011.07611.x.

Zhang, Y., B. Niu, D. Yu, X. Cheng, B. Liu, and J. Deng. 2010. "Radial glial cells and the lamination of the cerebellar cortex." Brain Struct Funct 215 (2):115-22. doi: 10.1007/s00429-010-0278-5.

Index

Note: *Italic* page numbers indicate figures.

A

Action potential, 138, 141–142
  in chemical synapse, *140, 143,* 153, *156*
  in electrical synapses, *145*
  and myelin disturbance, 201
Action potential speed (APS), 201
Activated microglial phase, 209, *210, 211*
Adenosine triphosphate (ATP), 198
Adipose tissue, 22
  and eyes, 233
  and PGI, *36*
  in spinal cord, *42*
  in spinal cord–fascia transition zone, *43*
Adrenal gland, *248*
Amniotic cavity, *107*
ANS, *see* Autonomic nervous system
Anterior spinal artery, 180
Anus, 253, *253*
APS (action potential speed), 201
Aquaporin(s), 79
  and BBB, *187*
  and CSF flow, 81, *82, 84, 95, 99*
  and CSF reabsorption pathways, 86, *89*
Aquaporin channels, 81, 93
Arachnoid membrane, 14, *15, 18,* 28
  and blood supply to brain, *181, 182*
  and bone-brain interconnection, *39*
  in CNS, *4*
  and CSF production/flow, 74, *76, 80,* 81, *82, 98*
  and CSF reabsorption pathways, *89, 96*
  and dural sac, *45*
  and dural venous sinus system, 21, *21*
  and dura mater meningeal layer, 22
  and fascial-glial network strain, *49, 50*
  and fascial strain transmission, *51, 52*
  infolding, 19–21, *20–22*
  and parenchymal capillaries, *77*
  and parenchymal strain transmission, *53, 54*
  and PGI, *36, 38*
  and SAV, *102*
  and spinal cord, 22, *23, 42, 43, 46*
  and subarachnoid space barrier, 30, *32*
Arachnoid trabecula, *15, 18, 23*
  and bone-brain interconnection, *39*
  and dural sac, *45*
  and fascial-glial network strain, *49, 50*
  and fascial strain transmission, *51, 52*
  and parenchymal strain transmission, *53, 54*
  and perineural CSF drainage pathway, *97*

287

and PGI, *38*
and SAV, *102*
and spinal cord, *42, 46*
spinal cord–fascia transition zone, *43*
Arachnoid villi (AV), 28
and CSF production/flow, 26, 63
and CSF reabsorption pathways, 88, *88, 90–92, 96, 101, 102*
and SAV, *102*
Area postrema, *189*
Arteries, *49, 50, 77, 181, 182*
Arterioles, 180, *182, 186*
Astrocyte(s), *37, 121–123, 126*
astrogliosis, 213–222, *214, 215, 217–222*
and BBB, 29, 185, *186*, 188
and biomechanical strain transmission, 48
and bone-brain interconnection, *39*
cell structure, 117, *118, 119*
and CNS function optimization, *151*, 154–155
and CSF flow, 58, *84, 99*
domain organization, 213, *214, 218, 219, 221*
dysregulation of, 223–225
and ECS, *131*, 165
and fascial strain transmission, *51, 52*
functions, 127, 223
and glial syncytium, 120–124, *121–123, 125*
and glia-neuron interaction, *137*
and gliotransmitters, *156*
glucose in, *149*
glutamate-glutamine shuttle, *151*
and interstitial blood flow regulation, *192*
and intracellular volume transmission, *176*
mini-domains, 124, *126*
and neural signaling, 146–147, *149–151*, 152–154
and neuron metabolism, 146–147, *149–151*
and neurovascular unit, 190, *191–193*
overview, 117–127, *118, 119, 121–123, 125, 126*
and parenchymal capillaries, *77*
and parenchymal strain transmission, *53, 54*
perivascular glial limiting membrane CSF, *95*
and PGI, 37, *38*
and potassium spatial buffering, *160*
and radial glia, 113
retinal, 231
SGCs *vs.*, 247
in spinal cord–fascia transition zone, *43*
synapses and, 130
in three-part synapse, *131*, 146–160, *148–151, 156–160*
and Virchow-Robin spaces, *83*
Astrocyte aquaporins, 79
Astrocyte calcium waves, *see* Calcium waves
Astrocyte channels, *119, 122*, 154–155, *187*
Astrocyte end-feet, *37*, 65, 117, *118, 119*, 120
arterioles and, 180
and BBB, *186, 187*
and bone-brain interconnection, *39*
and CNS capillaries, 185
and CSF production/flow, *73, 78, 82, 85, 89, 93*
and ECS shape, 165
and ependymal cells, *67, 73, 85*
and fascial-glial network strain, *49, 50*
and fascial strain transmission, *51, 52*

glucose transport, 147
glutamate-glutamine shuttle, *151*
and neural signaling, *150*
and outer glial limiting membrane, 29
and parenchymal capillaries, *77*
and parenchymal strain transmission, *53, 54*
and perinodal processes, *159*
and perivascular CSF flow, 81, *84*, 95
and PGI, 37, *38*
and potassium spatial buffering, *160*
and rootlet transition zone, *47*
in spinal cord–fascia transition zone, *43*
and synapses, 130
and synaptic stripping, 223
in three-part synapse, *131, 148*
and venule CSF flow, *99*
and Virchow-Robin spaces, *83*
Astrocyte end-feet channels, *73, 122*
Astrocyte gap junctions, *187*
Astrocyte matrix, 30, *77, 154, 202*
Astrocyte perinodal processes, *see* Perinodal processes
Astrocyte transporters, *187*
Astrogliosis, 213–222, *214, 215, 217–222*
ATP (adenosine triphosphate), 198
Autonomic nervous system (ANS), 74, 75, 247–252, *248–252*
AV, *see* Arachnoid villi
Axons, *196, 197*
and astrocyte perinodal processes, *159*
and dorsal root ganglion, 258, *261, 262*
and enteric ganglion, *256*
and enteric glia, *257*
and myelin, 195–198, *196, 197*
and myelinating Schwann cells, 238, *239*
in neural networks, *168*
in Neuron Doctrine, 132, *133*
and nodes of Ranvier, 199
and non-myelinating Schwann cells, *242*
and olfactory nerves, *263*
and perisynaptic Schwann cells, *243*
and potassium spatial buffering, *160*
and rootlet transition zone, *47*
and Schwann cell perinodal microvilli, *241*
and sympathetic/parasympathetic ganglia, *251, 252*
Wallerian degeneration, 243–246, *245, 246*

B

Bacterial receptors, *206*
Basal lamina, 65
and BBB, *186*
and bone-brain interconnection, *39*
and CSF capillary production, *78*
and CSF production/flow, *68, 73, 81, 82, 84, 85, 95, 99*
and CSF reabsorption pathways, *89*
and ependymal cells, *67*
and fascial-glial network strain, *49, 50*
and fascial strain transmission, *51, 52*
and parenchymal capillaries, *77*
and parenchymal strain transmission, *53, 54*
and PGI, 37, *38*
and rootlet transition zone, *47*
and Schwann cell perinodal microvilli, *241*
and Schwann cell potassium regulation, 240
spinal cord–fascia transition zone, *43*
and Virchow-Robin spaces, *83*

Basement membrane (BM), 183–184, *187*
Basic fibroblast growth factor, 212
BBB, *see* Blood-brain barrier
Biochemical transmission, 48
Biomechanical forces (BF), 48
Biomechanical shape (BS), 48
Biomechanical strain/stress, 33, *34, 41, 56,* 155, 225
Bipolar cell, *229*
Bladder, *248, 249*
Blastocoel, *107*
Blastocyst, *106, 107*
Blood, ependymal cell CSF and, 71
Blood-brain barrier (BBB), 29, 179–189, *181, 182, 186, 187, 189*
    areas without, 188, *189*
    components, 183–187, *186, 187*
    and glucose entering astrocyte, *149*
    and glucose transport, 147
    and parenchyma, 180–182, *181, 182*
    and pericytes, 185
    repair, 188
Blood-CSF barrier, 27, 29, 66
Blood flow, 190, *191–193,* 194
Blood plasma, 65
Blood vessels, *126*
    in brain, 188–189
    and ECS, *163*
    and enteric glia, *257*
    and glial cells in ECS, *167*
    and glial limiting membranes, *7, 31*
    and glucose entering astrocyte, *149*
    and Virchow-Robin spaces, *83*
BM (basement membrane), 183–184, 187
Bone
    and arachnoid villi CSF reabsorption pathway, *96*
    and blood supply to brain, *182*
    in CNS, *4*
    and fascial strain transmission, *51, 52*
    interconnection with glia, *3, 4*
    and meninges, 22, *24*
    and parenchymal capillaries, *77*
    and parenchymal strain transmission, *53, 54*
    and PGI, *38*
    and spinal cord, *42*
    spinal cord–fascia transition zone, *43*
    and subarachnoid space barrier, *32*
Bone marrow, *250*
Bony cranium, *62*
Bony orbit, 233
Brain, *15, 18, 24, 62*
    adult, *61*
    biomechanical strain transmission, *34, 35*
    blood flow requirements, 188
    blood supply to, 180, *181, 182,* 188–189
    CFS "floating" of, 59, *62*
    and CNS, *38*
    CSS maintenance and protection of, 13
    CVOs in, *189*
    and ECS, *164*
    embryonic, 59, *60, 111*
    encasing by meninges, 14, *18*
    and ephaptic coupling, *175*
    and EVT, *173*
    and intracellular volume transmission, *177*
    lateral view, *36*
    and parenchymal capillaries, *77*
    and PGI, *36*
    power generated by, 189, *189*
    quantity of neurons in, 132
    transition zone to fascia, *39*
    and ventricular system, *64*
    and wired transmission, *169*
Brain-derived neurotrophic factor, 212

Bruch's membrane, *235*
BS (biomechanical shape), 48

C

C2/C3 (dura mater membrane bony attachment), 22, *24*
Calcium channels, *143*
Calcium waves, 152, *158*, 171, *176*
Capillaries, 27
   and BBB, 183, *186*, *187*
   and blood supply to brain, *181*
   and CSF capillary production, 78
   and CSF production/flow, *69*, 84
   and neurovascular unit, *191*
   parenchymal, 77
   perivascular glial limiting membrane CSF, *95*
   and potassium spatial buffering, *160*
Cardiovascular system, 63
Carotid artery, 91, *100*, 180
Cavernous sinus, *21*
Cell body, *37*, *118*, *119*
Cell membrane, *123*
Central canal, 25, *28*, 65
   and CSF flow, *72*
   and spinal cord, *42*, *112*
   and ventricular system, *64*
Central nervous system (CNS)
   astrocytes and, 127, *151*, 154–155
   astrocyte matrix and, 30
   biomechanical strain transmission, *34*, *35*
   blood flow and basement membrane, 184
   causes of dysfunction, 3
   components, 1
   craniosacral system, *see* Craniosacral system (CSS)
   craniosacral therapy and CNS blood flow, 194
   CSF production in capillaries, 74, *77*, *78*
   and ECS, 162
   extracellular space in, 161–167, *163*, *164*, *167*
   fluid barriers, 27, 29–32, *31*, *32*
   glial cells in, 10, *12*
   interstitium, *See* Interstitium
   lateral view, *38*
   microglia's role in healing, 212
   neural tube and, *110*
   neurogenesis, 109, *111*, *112*, 113
   and neuro-glial-vascular interactions, 2
   and PGI, 37
   transmission within, 166–177, *167–169*, *172–177*
   Wallerian degeneration, 243, *246*
Cerebral aqueduct, 25, 63, *64*
Cerebral cortex, *116*, *200*
Cerebral hypertension, 59
Cerebrospinal fluid (CSF), 25–26, *28*, 57–102, *62*
   arachnoid membrane production of, 74, *76*
   classical model of production, 63
   CNS capillaries and, 74, *77*, *78*
   and CNS health, 25
   CSS distortion and, 92–94
   CST and, 3
   drainage (classical view), 26
   and dural venous sinus system, 21
   flow from ventricles into CNS tissue (classical view), 26
   glial regulation of circulation, 79–86, *80*, *82–86*
   importance of, 58–62, *60–62*
   production (classical view), 25, *28*
   production sites for, 63–78, *64*, *67–70*, *72*, *73*, *75–78*
   quantity/rate of renewal, 26
   reabsorption pathways, 86–92, *88*, *89*

stages of production, 66
total average adult amount, 63
ventricular system production of,
    63–74, *64, 67–70, 72, 73*
Cerebrovascular basement membrane,
    88, 91, *100*
Cervical lymphatics, 91, *250*
Channels, 120, *122, 123. See also
    specific channels*
Chemical synapses, 138–140, *139, 140*
Chemokines, 204, *206*
Choroidal vessels, *235*
Choroid plexus, *28, 60, 61*
    and ANS regulation of CSF, 74
    and CSF production/flow, 63,
        65–66, *68,* 81
    and CSF reabsorption, 66, *70*
    ependymal cells, 27, *28*
    and ventricular system, *64*
Chronic pain, 266
Cilia, 65, *67, 73*
Circumventricular organs (CVOs), 72,
    188, *189*
Cisterna magna, 79, *80*
CNS, *see* Central nervous system
CNS interstitium, *see* Interstitium
Coccyx, *15,* 22, *24*
Communication, neural, *see* Signaling;
    Transmission, CNS cell
Compact glial scar, 216, *219,* 220, *222,
    246*
Conduction, 132, *133*
Cones, 228, *229, 232*
Connexons, 120, *123*
Conus medullaris, 25. *See also* Spinal
    cord
Corpus callosum, *200*
Cranial arachnoid villi, *88,* 90, *96*
Cranial bones, *15,* 36
Cranial subarachnoid space, *28, 36, 72*
Craniosacral system (CSS), 13–32,
    15–21, 23, 24, 28, 31, 32
    astrocyte matrix and, 30
    bones attached to meninges, 22, *24*
    cerebrospinal fluid, 25–26, *28*
    choroid plexus ependymal cells, 27,
        28
    and CNS, 27, 29–32, *31, 32*
    and CSF dynamics, 92–94
    functions, 1
    glial cells in, 26–27
    infolding of dura mater/arachnoid
        membranes, *19–21,* 19–22
    meninges, 14–20, *15–20,* 22, *24*
    ventricular system ependymal cells,
        27, *28*
Craniosacral therapy (CST)
    basement membrane and, 184
    and CNS blood flow, 194
    to correct myelin disturbances, 202
    and ECS shape, 166
    and eye health, 233–234
    and fascial-glial strain correction, *50*
    for head trauma, 224–225
    lessening of and astrocyte stress by,
        155
    and pia-glial interface, 3
    and PNS glia, 265–267
    potential benefits, 267
    primary goals of, 2–3
Cribriform plate, 90, *97, 263*
Critical diameter, 198
CSF, *see* Cerebrospinal fluid
CSS, *see* Craniosacral system
CST, *see* Craniosacral therapy
CVOs, *see* Circumventricular organs
Cyst, *222*
Cytokines, 204, *206*

D

Debris removal
    by astrocytes, 213
    and astrogliosis, *215, 217–219*
    and CST, 224

by microglia, *206,* 207, *208,* 209, 212
Dendrites, 132, *133,* 135, 212
Denticulate ligament, *23, 42, 102*
Differentiation, 104
Diffuse astrogliosis, 216, *218*
Direct channel receptor, 142
Domain organization, 213, *214, 218, 219, 221*
Dorsal ramus, *260*
Dorsal root, *40, 44, 46, 102*
Dorsal root ganglia (DRG), 258–262, *259–262*
    and dural sac, *45*
    and PGI, *40*
    and radicular veins, *101*
    and SAV, *102*
    and spinal cord, *46*
Dorsal root ganglion satellite glia, *262*
Dorsal rootlet, *44, 46, 102*
Drainage, CSF, 26
DRG, *see* Dorsal root ganglia
Dural sac, *15–17, 45, 46, 101, 259, 261*
Dural venous sinus system, 21, *21*
    and classical model of CSF production, 63
    and CSF drainage, 26
    and CSF reabsorption pathways, 86, 90, 91, *96*
Dura mater membrane, *15, 18,* 22, *24,* 28
    and blood supply to brain, *181, 182*
    and bone-brain interconnection, *39*
    in CNS, *4*
    and CSF production/flow, *76, 80, 82, 97*
    and CSF reabsorption pathways, *89, 96*
    and dural sac, *45*
    and dural venous sinus system, 21
    and fascial-glial network strain, *49, 50*
    and fascial strain transmission, *51, 52*
    infolding, *19–21,* 19–22
    and parenchymal capillaries, *77*
    and parenchymal strain transmission, *53, 54*
    and PGI, *36, 38*
    and SAV, *102*
    and spinal cord, *42, 46*
    spinal cord–fascia transition zone, *43*
    and subarachnoid space barrier, 30, *32*
    trabeculae, 14
Dura mater meningeal layer, 22, *23*
Dura mater priosteal layer, 22
Dystrophic microglial phase, 209, *211*

E

ECM, *see* Extracellular matrix
ECM ground substance, 48
ECS, *see* Extracellular space
Ectoderm, *107, 110, 238*
Ectodermal cell differentiation, 104
Electrical fields, ephaptic coupling and, 170–171, *174, 175*
Electrical synapses, *139,* 144, *145*
Embryo, *238*
Embryoblast, *107*
Embryonic mesoderm, 204
Embryonic period, 104–105, *107*
End branch, 132, *133*
End-feet, *See* Astrocyte end-feet
Endoderm, *107, 238*
Endodermal cell differentiation, 105
Endoneurium, *98*
Endothelial cells, *78,* 183–185, *187*
Endothelium, *100,* 185
Energy substrate, *150*
Enteric ganglion, *256*

Enteric glia, *253*, 253–257, *254, 256, 257*
Enteric nervous system (ENS), *253*, 253–257, *254, 256, 257*
Ependymal cells, 28, 65, *126*
   and choroid plexus, 27, 28, 65–66
   and choroid plexus CSF reabsorption, 66, *70*
   and CSF production/flow, *68, 69, 71, 73*, 85, *85*
   and ventricular system, 27, *28, 64*
   and ventricular system CSF, 63
Ephaptic coupling, 170–171, *174, 175*
Epidural space, 22, *23, 36, 40, 42, 43*
ESN (excess synaptic neurotransmitter), 154–155
Esophagus, *253*
Evolution, myelin and, 199
Excess synaptic neurotransmitter (ESN), 154–155
Excitatory response, 138, *140*
Extracellular matrix (ECM)
   and astrocyte release of gliotransmitters, *156*
   and astrocyte stimulated by neurotransmitter, *157*
   and basement membrane, 183
   and biomechanical strain transmission, 48
   and bone-brain interconnection, *39*
   and dorsal root ganglion, *262*
   and fascial strain transmission, *51, 52*
   and parenchymal strain transmission, *53, 54*
   and PGI, *38*
   and spinal cord–fascia transition zone, *43*
   and sympathetic/parasympathetic ganglia, *252*

Extracellular space (ECS), *122, 123, 131*, 161–167, *163, 164, 167*
   astrocytes and, 127
   and bone-brain interconnection, *39*
   cleansing of, 79
   as CNS passageway, 165
   ECM molecules and, 162
   and ephaptic coupling, *174*
   and EVT, 170, *172*
   and glia, 165–166, *167*
   and glial syncytium, *125*
   and glucose entering astrocyte, *149*
   glutamate-glutamine shuttle, *151*
   and intracellular volume transmission, *176*
   and myelination, 198
   and neural signaling, *150*
   and PGI, *38*
   and potassium spatial buffering, 153, *160*
   synapses and, 130
Extracellular volume transmission (EVT), 170, *172, 173*
Eye(s), *228, 229*
   CST and, 233–234
   parasympathetic division of ANS, *249*
   retinal glia, 227–235, *228, 229, 232, 235*
   and RPE, *235*
   sympathetic division of ANS, *248*
Eyelids, 233–234
Eye muscles, 233

F

Fallopian tubes, *106*
Falx cerebelli, 19, *20*
Falx cerebri, 19, *19, 20*

Fascia
- and basement membrane, 184
- biomechanical strain transmission, *35,* 48
- and CST, 265
- disturbances of, 48
- and dorsal root ganglion, *262*
- and enteric ganglion, *256*
- and enteric glia, *257*
- and fascial-glial matrix adverse strain, *41*
- and fascial-glial network strain, *49*
- and fascial strain transmission, *51*
- and parenchyma, 33–36, *34–36*
- and PGI, *36,* 37, *40*
- and SAV, *102*
- and spinal cord, *42, 46*
- sympathetic/parasympathetic ganglia, *252*
- transmission of biomechanical strain, *34*
- transmission zone to brain, *39*

Fascial-glial matrix, *41*
Fascial-glial network strain, *49*
Fascial layers, 14
Fascial matrix, 184, 266
Fascial patterns, 184
Fascial strain transmission, *51*
Fenestrated capillaries, 65, *68*
Fetal period, 108, *108*
Fibroblasts, 14, 74, *257*
Fibrous astrocytes, *118*
Fibrous proteins, 48
Filum terminale externum, *15*
Fluid barriers, 27, 29–32, *31, 32.* See also *specific barriers; specific membranes*
Foramen magnum, 22, *24*
Foramen of Luschka, 71

Foramen of Magendie, 71, *72*
Foramen of Monro, 25, 63, *64*
Fourth ventricle, 25, 26, *28,* 65
- and CSF flow, 71, *72*
- and ependymal cells, *67*
- and ventricular system, *64*

G

Gallbladder, *248, 249*
Gamma aminobutyric acid (GABA), 147
Ganglia
- and ANS, 247
- parasympathetic division of ANS, *249*
- in retina, *229*
- sympathetic division of ANS, *248*
- sympathetic/parasympathetic, *251*
- sympathetic/parasympathetic innervation of immune organs, *250*

Gap junctions, 136, 138
- and astrocyte perinodal processes, *159*
- and BBB, *187*
- and dorsal root ganglion satellite glia, *262*
- in electrical synapses, *139,* 144, *145*
- glial, 120, *122, 123*
- and glial syncytium, 152
- and glucose entering astrocyte, *149*
- and intracellular volume transmission, *176*
- and potassium spatial buffering, *160*
- and sympathetic/parasympathetic ganglia, *252*

Gastrointestinal (GI) tract, *253,* 253–256
Gastrula, *107*
Genitalia, *248, 249*
Germ cell layers, 104

Germinal neuroepithelial cells, 58
GI (gastrointestinal) tract, 253, 253–256
Glia. See also specific glia, e.g., Retinal glia
   about, 9–11, *12*
   in CNS, *4,* 10, *12*
   and CSF physiology, 57
   in CSS, 26–27
   and CSS/CNS interconnection, 30
   and ECS, *163,* 165–166, *167*
   and ephaptic coupling, *174*
   and EVT, *172*
   functions, 1, 10–12, *12*
   interconnection with bones, 3, *4*
   inter-workings with neurons, 136, *137*
   and neurons, 2–3
   new discoveries about, 135–136
   peripheral nervous system glia, 11, *12*
   regulation of CSF circulation, 79–86, *80, 82–86*
Glial cell-derived neurotrophic factor, 212
Glial gap junctions, 120, *122, 123*
Glial limiting membranes, 5–6
   inner, *see* Inner glial limiting membrane
   outer, *see* Outer glial limiting membrane
   perivascular, *see* Perivascular glial limiting membrane
Glial matrix, *4*
Glial neurotransmitter receptors, 152, *157*
Glial syncytium, 48, *54,* 120–124, *121–123, 125,* 152–154
Gliosis, 203. *See also* Astrogliosis
Gliotransmitters, 152, 154, *156*

Glomerulus, *263*
Glossopharyngeal nerve, 75
Glucose, 146–147, *149,* 188
Glucose transporter, *149*
Glutamate, 141, 147, *151*
Glutamate-glutamine shuttle, *151*
Glutamine, *151*
Glycogen, 147, *150*
Glycosaminoglycans, 162
Glymphatic system, 79–80, *80*
Golgi, Camillo, 130–131
Gray matter, *118*
Growth factors, CSF, 58

H

Head trauma, 224
Heart, *248, 249*
Homeostasis, 179
Hydrocephalus, 59

I

Immune cells, 231, *257*
Immune response, 204
Indirect channel receptor, 142
Inferior sagittal sinus, *21*
Inflammation, 165–166, 220, 224
Inhibitory response, 138, *140, 143, 145*
Inner glial limiting membrane, 6, *7,* 29, *31, 67, 85*
Internodes, 238
Interstitial blood flow, *192, 193*
Interstitial fluid (ISF), 79, 86, 92
Interstitium, 6, *7*
   and BBB, 29, 185, 190
   and CSF flow, *80, 82, 84, 85,* 99
   and CSF reabsorption pathways, *89, 92*
   and glial limiting membrane, *31*

glucose in, 146–147
perivascular glial limiting membrane
   CSF, 95
and SAV, 102
and subarachnoid space barrier, 32
Interventricular foramina, 25. *See also*
   Foramen of Monro
Intervertebral foramina, 43
Intestines, 248, 249, 253, 253–256,
   254
Intracellular communication, 152
Intracellular space, 122, 123
Intracellular volume transmission, 171,
   176, 177
Ion(s), 135, 144, 145, 231
Ion channels, 135, 142, 144, 204
Ionotropic receptor, 142
ISF, *see* Interstitial fluid

J

Jugular veins, 26, 88

K

Kidney, 248

L

Lacrimal gland, 249
Lactate, 146, 147, 150
Large intestine, 253, 253, 254
Lateral ventricles, 25, 28, 61, 65
   and CSF flow, 72
   and ependymal cells, 67
   and ventricular system, 64
Light transmission by Muller cells, 231,
   232
Liver, 248, 249
Lumen
   artery, 100

capillary, 187
neural tube, 58, 59
small intestine, 254
Lungs, 248, 249
Lymphatic system, 90, 91
Lymphoid tissue, 250

M

Macrocircuits, 132
Median eminence, 189
Membrane channel, 66, 69, 70
Meningeal layer (dura mater
   membrane), 14, 18, 39, 43, 80
Meningeal sheath, 233
Meningeal stress, 194, 224
Meninges, 14–20, 15–20, 24, 39
   and arachnoid membrane CSF
      production, 76
   arachnoid membrane infolding, 19,
      19, 20
   biomechanical strain transmission,
      34, 35
   bones attached to, 22, 24
   cell structure, 14
   dura mater membrane infolding,
      19–21, 19–22
   encasing of brain by, 14, 18
   spinal cord encasement, 22, 23
Mesoderm, 107, 238
Mesodermal cells, differentiation of,
   105
Metabotropic receptor, 144
Microcircuits, 132
Micro-domains, 136
Microglia, 124, 204–213, 205, 206,
   208, 210, 211
   and CNS healing, 212
   critical functions of, 223
   dysregulation of, 223–225
   micro-domains, 204, 205
   and neural plasticity, 212
   receptors, 204, 206, 207

retinal, 231
states, 207–211, *208, 210, 211*
and synapse formation, 212–213
Microglial stripping, 223
Microgliosis, 209, *221*. See also Activated microglial phase
Micro-regions, 190
Micro-vessel flow, 188
Microvilli, 65, 233, 240, *241*
Mid-line ganglion, *248*
Midsagittal section of brain, *39*
Mild astrogliosis, 213, *215*
Mini-domains, astrocyte, 124, *126*
Mitral cell, *263*
Moderate astrogliosis, 216, *217*
Morula, *106*
Motor neurons, *49, 50*
Mucosa, *254*
Mucosal glia, 254, 255
Muller cells, 227, *228, 229,* 230–231, *232*
Muscle fibers, *243*
Myelin, *126*
    and astrocyte perinodal processes, *159*
    disturbance of, 201–202
    and dorsal root ganglia, *261, 262*
    and microglia, 212
    and myelinating Schwann cells, *239*
    and non-myelinating Schwann cells, *242*
    and oligodendrocytes, 195–200, *196, 197, 199, 200*
    and potassium spatial buffering, 153, *160*
    and rootlet transition zone, *47*
    and Schwann cell perinodal microvilli, *241*
    and sympathetic/parasympathetic ganglia, *252*
    and Wallerian degeneration, *245, 246*
Myelinated nerve fiber rootlet transition zone, *47*
Myelinating Schwann cells, 238, *239*
Myelination, *196,* 196–198, *197*
Myenteric plexus, *254*
Myofibroblasts, 255

N

Nerve cell body, *251, 252, 256, 257, 262*
Nerve growth factor, 212
Nerve roots, *15–17, 23, 41*
Nervous system development
    central nervous system neurogenesis, 109, *111, 112,* 113
    peripheral nervous system neurogenesis, *110,* 113
    radial glia and, 109–116, *110–112, 114–116*
Neural conduction, 132, *133*
Neural crest cells, *110,* 113, 237, *238*
Neural dysfunction, 154
Neural groove, *110*
Neural networks, *134, 168*
Neural plasticity, 212
Neural plate, *110*
Neural signaling, *see* Signaling
Neural tube, 58, *110, 238*
Neuroactive substances, 170
Neuroepithelial cells, 109
Neurogenesis, 109, *110–112,* 113
Neurohormone receptors, *206*
Neurological signaling, 198, 199
Neuromodulators, 130
Neuron(s), *126, 133,* 199
    about, 9
    and astrocyte matrix, 154
    and astrocyte perinodal processes, *159*
    dying, 212
    in ECS, *131, 163, 167*
    in ENS, 254

and ephaptic coupling, *174*
and EVT, 170, *172*
generation during fetal
  development, 59
and glia, 2–3, *167*
inter-workings with glia, 136, *137*
linkage to BBB, 190
metabolic support, 146–147,
  149–151
migration along radial glia, 109,
  113, *114–116*
in neural networks, *134, 168*
and neural signaling design, 201
new discoveries about, 135
nutrient requirements, 188
and potassium spatial buffering, 153
quantity in brain, 132
and radial glia, *114*
and three-part synapse, *148*
and two-part synapse model, 130–
  145, *133, 134, 137, 139, 140,
  143, 145*
and vision, 228
Neuron Doctrine, 130–137, *133, 134,
  137*
Neuropeptides, 141
Neurotransmitter(s), *140,* 141
  and astrocyte release of
    gliotransmitters, *156*
  astrocytes stimulated by, *157*
  astrocytes' uptake of, 154
  in chemical synapses, 138, *140, 143*
  and ECS shape, 165
  and interstitial blood flow
    regulation, *192*
  receptor channels, 142, 144
  in two-part synapses, 129
Neurotransmitter receptors, *206*
Neurotransmitter substrate, *151*
Neurovascular unit, 179, 188–193, *189,
  191–193*
NG-2 cells, 124
Nitric oxide, 71–72

Nodes of Ranvier, 199, *199*
  and astrocyte perinodal processes,
    159
  and myelinating Schwann cells, 238,
    239
  potassium regulation at, 153–154,
    240, 241
  and potassium spatial buffering, *160*
  and Schwann cell perinodal
    microvilli, *241*
Nodose ganglia, 258
Non-myelinated nerve fiber rootlet
  transition zone, *47*
Non-myelinating Schwann cells, 240,
  242
Nutrients, CNS cell, 188

O

Occipital sinus, *21*
Olfactory bulb, *97, 263*
Olfactory ensheathing glia (OEG), *98,
  263,* 264
Olfactory epithelium, *97, 263*
Olfactory nerves, *97, 98, 263*
Olfactory neural precursor cells, 264
Olfactory perineural channel, *88*
Olfactory receptor neuron, *263,* 264
Oligodendrocytes, *126,* 136
  and myelin disturbance, 201–202
  and myelin production/
    maintenance, 195–200, *196, 197,
    199, 200*
One-to-many communication, 170.
  See also Ephaptic coupling;
  Extracellular volume transmission;
  Intracellular volume transmission
One-to-one communication, 166. *See
  also* Wired transmission
Organs (CVOs), 188

Organum vasculosum of the lamina terminalis, *189*
Outer glial limiting membrane, 5, *7, 29, 31*
   arterioles and, 180
   and blood supply to brain, *182*
   and bone-brain interconnection, *39*
   and CSF reabsorption, 87, *89*
   and fascial-glial strain correction, *50*
   and head trauma, 224
   and PGI, 37, *38*
   and pia mater membrane CSF flow, *82*
   and spinal cord, *46*
   spinal cord–fascia transition zone, *43*
   spinal cord rootlet transition zone, *44*
   and subarachnoid space barrier, *32*
Ovary, *106, 248, 249*
Ovum, *106*
Oxygen, 188

P

Pain
   CST for control of, 266–267
   perception of, 141
   PNS glial disturbance and, 264–266
Pancreas, *248, 249*
Parasympathetic division satellite glia, 247, *249–252*
Parasympathetic innervation, 74, *75*, 250
Parenchyma
   about, 4, 5
   and astrocyte-adverse biomechanical stress, 155
   and BBB, 180–182, *181, 182, 186*
   and blood supply to brain, *181*
   in CNS, 5
   and CSF drainage pathway, *97*
   and CSF production/flow, 26, 59, 63, 71, *76*
   and fascia, 33–36, *34–36*
   and fascial-glial network strain, *49*
   and Virchow-Robin spaces, *83*
Parenchymal strain transmission, 53
Parotid gland, *248, 249*
Pathogens, *206, 208, 215, 219*
Pattern-recognition receptors, 204
Pericytes, *78*, 184–185, *187*
Perineural space, 90–91, *97, 98*
Perinodal microvilli, 240, *241*
Perinodal processes, 153–154, *159, 160*
Periosteal layer (dura mater membrane), 14, *18*, 22, *39*
Peripheral nervous system (PNS)
   neurogenesis, *110*, 113
   Wallerian degeneration, 243, *245*
Peripheral nervous system (PNS) glia, 11, *12*, 237–267
   CST and, 265–267
   dysfunction, 264–265
   enteric, *253*, 253–257, *254, 256, 257*
   olfactory ensheathing glia, *263*, 264
   Schwann cells, 238–246, *239, 241–243, 245–246*
   sympathetic/parasympathetic division satellite glia, 247–252, *248–252*
Perisynaptic Schwann cells, 240, *243*
Perivascular channels, *100*
Perivascular glial limiting membrane, 6, *7, 29, 31*
   and BBB, *186, 187*
   and blood supply to brain, *182*
   and CSF flow, 81
   and CSF reabsorption, 86, 90, 91, *95*
   and Virchow-Robin spaces, *83*
Perivascular space
   and BBB, *186, 187*
   and blood supply to brain, *182*

and choroid plexus CSF
  reabsorption, 66, *70*
and CNS capillary CSF, 74
and CSF capillary production, 78
and CSF production/flow, 68, 69,
  80, 81, *83*, *84*
and glial cells in ECS, *167*
and glucose entering astrocyte, *149*
and parenchymal capillaries, 77
perivascular glial limiting membrane
  CSF, 95
and Virchow-Robin spaces, *83*
Petrosal sinus, *21*
Phospholipids, *196*, *197*
Photoreceptors, 228, 233
Pia-glial interface (PGI), 33–56, *38–47*,
  49–56
  and astrocyte-adverse biomechanical
    stress, 155
  and biochemical transmission, 48
  and biomechanical adverse strain
    patterns, 56
  and bone-brain interconnection, *39*
  as corrective interface, 48–56,
    49–56
  and CST, 202
  and fascial-glial network strain, *49*,
    50
  and fascial strain transmission, *51*,
    52
  movement of forces in, 37–47,
    38–47
  and parenchymal strain
    transmission, *53*, *54*
Pia mater membrane, *7*, 14, *18*, *23*, 28,
  126
  arterioles and, 180
  and blood supply to brain, *181*, *182*
  and bone-brain interconnection, *39*
  in CNS, *4*, *5*
  and CSF production/flow, 26, *76*,
    80, 81, *82*, *97*, *98*

and CSF reabsorption pathways, 87,
  89, 96
in developing brain, *111*
in developing spinal cord, *112*
and dural sac, *45*
and fascial-glial network strain, *49*,
  50
and fascial strain transmission, *52*
and head trauma, 224
and migrating neurons, *116*
and parenchymal capillaries, 77
and parenchymal strain
  transmission, *53*, *54*
and PGI, *36*, *37*, *38*
and radial glia, 109, *114*
and SAV, *102*
and spinal cord, 22, *42*, *46*
spinal cord–fascia transition zone,
  43
spinal cord rootlet transition zone,
  44
and subarachnoid space barriers,
  29–30
and Virchow-Robin spaces, *83*
Pineal gland, *189*
Pituitary gland, *189*
PNS, *see* Peripheral nervous system
Posterior spinal artery, 180
Postsynaptic folds, *243*
Postsynaptic neurons, *130*, 142
  and astrocyte stimulated by
    neurotransmitter, *157*
  in chemical synapse, *140*, *143*
  in chemical synapses, 138
  in synapse, *139*
  in three-part synapse, *131*, 146, *148*
Potassium channels, 153–154
Potassium regulation, Schwann cell,
  240, *241*
Potassium spatial buffering, 153–154,
  159, *160*
Precursor cells, 136, 264
Pre-embryonic period, 104, *106*

301

Prenatal development, 103–108, *106–108*
Pressure, CSF, 59
Presynaptic neuron, *130, 139*
   and astrocyte stimulated by neurotransmitter, *157*
   in chemical synapses, 138, *140, 143*
   in three-part synapse, *131,* 146, *148*
Protoplasmic astrocytes, *118*

R

Radial glia, 103–116, *106–108, 110–112, 114–116*
   about, 109, *111, 112*
   and nervous system development, 109–116, *110–112, 114–116*
   and prenatal development, 103–108, *106–108, 111, 112*
Radial migration, 109
Radicular veins, 92, *101*
Rami communicantes, *260*
Ramón y Cajal, Santiago, 130–131
Reabsorption of CSF, *see under* Cerebrospinal fluid (CSF), reabsorption pathways
Reactive astrogliosis with compact glial scar, 216, *219–222,* 220
Rectum, *248, 249, 253*
Resting microglial state, *208,* 211
Reticular theory, 131
Retina, 228, *229, 232*
Retinal astrocytes, 231
Retinal glia, 227–235, *228, 229, 232, 235*
   Muller cells, *228,* 230–231, *232*
   retinal astrocytes, 231
   retinal microglia, 231
   retinal pigment epithelium, 233, *235*
Retinal microglia, 231

Retinal pigment epithelium (RPE), 233, *235*
Rods, 228, *229, 232*
Rootlet transition zone, *46, 47*
Rostral migratory stream, 264

S

S2 (dura mater membrane bony attachment), *15,* 22, *24*
Sacrum, *15*
Satellite glial cells (SGCs), 258, *261, 262*
   common functions, 258
   and dorsal root ganglion, *262*
   sympathetic/parasympathetic division, 247–252, *248–252*
SAV, *see* Spinal arachnoid villi
Schwann cell(s), 238–246, *239, 241–243, 245–246*
   myelinating, 238, *239*
   non-myelinating, 240, *242*
   perisynaptic, 240, *243*
   potassium regulation, 240, *241*
   Wallerian degeneration, 243–246, *245, 246*
Schwann cell perinodal microvilli, 240, *241*
Sclera, 233
Sensory neurons, *49, 50*
Sensory system satellite glia, 258–262, *259–262*
Serosa, *254*
SGCs, *see* Satellite glial cells
Sigmoid sinus, *21*
Signaling. *See also* Neuron(s); Neurotransmitter(s); Synapses; Transmission, CNS cell
   astrocyte calcium waves, *158*
   astrocytes' role in, 130, 146–160, *149–151*
   by dying neurons, 212

by endothelial cells, 185
glial cells and, 10, 135, 136
and microglia, 204, 212
and microglial stripping, 223
myelin and, 195, 198, 201
myelinating Schwann cells, 238
in Neuron Doctrine, 132, 135
nitric oxide as medium for, 71–72
of pain, 266
retinal glia and, 227, 228
Schwann cells and, 238, 240
somatic sensory, 258
Skin, CST and, 265
Small intestine, 248, 249, 253, *253*, *254*, *256*
Small-molecule neurotransmitters, 141
S-nitrosoglutathione, 188
Sodium, 153
Soma, 132, *133*
Somatic sensory system, 258
Spatial buffering, 124
Sphenoparietal sinus, *21*
Spinal arachnoid villi (SAV), 88, 91–92, *101*, *102*
Spinal canal, 23, *42*, *43*
Spinal cord, 15, 23, *46*, 260
    biomechanical strain transmission, *35*
    blood supply to, 180
    CSS maintenance and protection of, 13
    and dural sac, *45*
    embryonic, *112*
    and ephaptic coupling, *175*
    and EVT, *173*
    and fascial-glial matrix adverse strain, *41*
    and intracellular volume transmission, *177*
    lateral view, *36*
    meninges' encasement of, 22, *23*
    and PGI, *36*
    and rootlet transition zone, *47*
    and SAV, *102*
    and ventricular system, *64*
    and wired transmission, *169*
Spinal cord gray matter, 23, 40, *42–44*, 260
Spinal cord rootlet transition zone, 44
Spinal cord white matter, 23, 40, *42–44*, 260
Spinal nerve, 40, *46*, 259, 260
Spinal subarachnoid space, 28, *36*, 72
Spleen, 248
Stomach, 248, 249, 253
Straight sinus, *21*
Stress, 37, 233. *See also* Biomechanical strain/stress; Meningeal stress
Subarachnoid space, 14, *15*, *18*, 23, 62
    and arachnoid membrane CSF production, *76*
    arteries in, 180
    and blood supply to brain, *181*, *182*
    and bone-brain interconnection, *39*
    and CSF, 26, 71, *72*, 79, *80*, 81, *82*, 97
    and CSF reabsorption pathways, *89*, 90
    and dural sac, *45*
    and fascial-glial network strain, *49*, *50*
    and glial limiting membrane, *31*
    and parenchymal capillaries, *77*
    and PGI, *38*
    and SAV, *102*
    and spinal cord, *42*, *46*
    spinal cord–fascia transition zone, *43*
    and subarachnoid space barrier, *32*
    and Virchow-Robin spaces, *83*
Subarachnoid space barriers, 29–30, 32
Subcommissural organ, *189*
Subfornical organ, *189*
Submaxillary gland, *249*
Submucosa, *254*

Submucosal plexus, *254*
Substance P, 141
Substantia alba, 196, *200*. *See also* Myelin
Subventricular zone, 58, *60, 61*
Superior cervical sympathetic ganglion, *75, 248*
Superior sagittal dural venous sinus, *96*
Superior sagittal sinus, *21, 28*
Surveillance state, 207, *208, 210, 211*
Swelling, 165–166
Sympathetic division satellite glia, 247, *248, 250–252*
Sympathetic ganglion, *40, 260*
Sympathetic innervation, 74, *75, 250*
Synapses, *126*
   and astrocyte release of gliotransmitters, *156*
   and astrocyte stimulated by neurotransmitter, *157*
   chemical, 138–140, *139, 140*
   components, 129–131, *130, 131*
   dysfunction of, 223
   electrical, *139*, 144, *145*
   and enteric glia, *257*
   and microglia, 212–213
   and neurovascular unit, *191*
   and Schwann cells, 240, *243*
   sympathetic/parasympathetic ganglia, *252*
   three-part, 130, *131*, 146–160, *148–151, 156–160*
   two-part, *see* Two-part synapses
   types of, 138–145, *139, 140, 143, 145*
Synaptic bouton, 141, 142
Synaptic cleft, *130*, 138, 142
   astrocytes' uptake of neurotransmitters in, 154
   in chemical synapse, *139, 140, 143*
   and ECS shape, 165

glial neurotransmitter receptor activation, 152
   in three-part synapse, *131, 148*
Synaptic signaling, *158*. *See also* Signaling
Synaptic stripping, 212, 223
Synaptogenesis, 213
Syncytium, 136

T

Tangential migration, 109
Tanycytes, 71–72, 188
Tentorium cerebelli, 19, *19, 20*
Third ventricle, 25, *28, 60, 61*, 65
   and CSF flow, *72*
   and ependymal cells, *67*
   and ventricular system, *64*
Three-part synapse, 130, *131*, 146–160, *148–151, 156–160*
Thrombospondins (TSPs), 212–213
Thymus, *250*
Tight junctions, 183, *187*
Timing, neural communication, 198, 201
Tonsils, *250*
Trabeculae, 14
Trachea, *248, 249*
Tracts (axon bundles), 198
Transmembrane protein, *69, 70*
Transmission, CNS cell, 166–177, *167–169, 172–177*
   ephaptic coupling, 170–171, *174, 175*
   extracellular volume, 170, *172, 173*
   intracellular volume, 171, *176, 177*
   wired, 166, *168, 169*
Transverse sinus, *21, 28*
Trigeminal ganglia, 258
Tripartite synapse, 146. *See also* Three-part synapse
Trophoblast, *107*

TSPs (thrombospondins), 212–213
Tunica adventitia, *100*
Two-part synapses, 129–131, *130, 131*
  elements of, 141–143, *143*
  Neuron Doctrine and, 130–137, *133, 134, 137*
  neurons and, 130–145, *133, 134, 137, 139, 140, 143, 145*

U

Uterus, *106, 248, 249*

V

Vagus nerve, *75*
Veins, *49, 50,* 91
Venous capillaries, *70. See also* Venules
Ventral ramus, *260*
Ventral root, *40, 44, 46, 102*
Ventral rootlet, *44, 46*
Ventricles. *See also specific ventricles, e.g.:*, Fourth ventricle
  CSF production/flow, 25, 26, 65, *67*
  in developing brain, *111*
  and ependymal cell CSF production, *73*
  ependymal cells in, 27, *28*
  and radial glia, 109, *114*
Ventricular cavity, 58, 66
  and choroid plexus CSF reabsorption, *70*
  and CSF production/flow, *68, 69, 73, 85*
  and ependymal cells, *67*
Ventricular system, *7, 28*
  and ANS regulation of CSF, *75*
  and ependymal cells, 27, *28*
  and glial limiting membrane, *31*
Ventricular system CSF production, 63–74, *64, 67–70, 72, 73*
  ANS regulation of, 74, *75*

choroid plexus CSF production, 65–66, *68*
choroid plexus CSF reabsorption, 66, *70*
ependymal cell CSF, 71, *73*
tanycytes, 71–72
ventricular flow into subarachnoid space, 71, *72*
Ventricular zone, 58, *60, 114*
Venules, *70,* 87, *88,* 91, *99*
Vertebra, *40*
Vertebral arch, *23*
Vertebral artery, 91, *100,* 180
Vertebral body, *23, 260*
Vertebral column, *41, 260*
Vesicles, 138, *140, 143*
Vesicular membrane, 142
Viral receptors, *206*
Virchow-Robin spaces, 81, *83,* 180, *181, 182*
Vision, *See* Eye(s)
Vitalizing (trophic) factors, 58

W

Wallerian degeneration, 243–246, *245, 246*
Water, ECS shape and, 165
Water content, of ISF and CSF, 86
White matter, *118,* 196. *See also* Myelin; Spinal cord white matter
Wired transmission, 166, *168, 169*

Y

Yoke sac, *107*

Z

Zygote, *106*

Other Products Available through Upledger Institute International

by Tad Wanveer, LMT, CST-D,
Certified Upledger Institute International Instructor

DVD: *In Motion - An Animated Exploration of the Craniosacral Rhythm*

Booklet: *CST Touching The Brain 1 (CTTB1) Symbols*

Chart: *Fascia; The Interwoven Body Wall Chart*

Courses: *CST Touching The Brain 1; Stimulating Self-Correction Through the Glial Interface (CTTB1)*
CST Touching The Brain 2; Stimulating Self-Correction Through the Glial Interface (CTTB2)

Titles of Related Interest

An Answer to Your Pain; CranioSacral Therapy for Health and Healing

A Brain Is Born; Exploring the Birth and Development of the Central Nervous System

Cell Talk; Transmitting Mind into DNA

CranioSacral Therapy; Touchstone for Natural Healing

It's All in the Gut; Let Your Second Brain Guide You to Optimal Health

Respectful Collaboration; Ten Clients, a Physician, and a CranioSacral Therapist—Inspiring Healings

SomatoEmotional Release and Beyond

SomatoEmotional Release; Deciphering the Language of Life

A Touch Better; Two Therapists' Journey and the Lessons They Learned from Dr. John E. Upledger about CranioSacral Therapy

Working Wonders; Changing Lives with CranioSacral Therapy

Your Inner Physician and You; CranioSacral Therapy and SomatoEmotional Release

Upledger Productions
Your source for educational excellence.

www.Upledger.com

Welcome
to Upledger Institute International

Upledger Institute International is a member of the International Alliance of Healthcare Educators (IAHE). When you study with IAHE you gain a lifelong resource for exceptional continuing education and professional support. With every course taken, you can be assured of our commitment to provide the highest level of instruction and service.

IAHE benefits include:

- Curriculums designed by the modality developer or top leaders in their field
- Classes taught by practicing healthcare professionals who have completed extensive teaching apprenticeship programs
- Seminars designed to enable you to begin confidently utilizing what you have learned with clients
- Contact hours to satisfy many cases of continuing-education unit (CEU) requirements
- Certificate of Attendance and CEU letter provided on the last day of class
- Networking with colleagues in class and beyond—class roster e-mailed to you within a few weeks following class
- Certification programs valued and recognized worldwide
- Reduced tuition for course review
- Workshops in more than 400 cities and 60 countries
- Access to study groups
- Personal online account for accessing transaction receipts
- Skilled educational-services counselors to assist you in registering for workshops, selecting products, and providing general information
- Access to a wide array of support material containing valuable insights into new research, techniques, and best practices
- Free membership through the International Association of Healthcare Practitioners (IAHP)
- Eligibility to upgrade to IAHP Medallion Membership, with benefits that include access to online video class review material, enhanced status on iahp.com referral site, a customized online therapist profile, and unlimited access to rosters of classes you've attended

We look forward to seeing you at an Upledger Institute International seminar – an exceptional learning and professional development experience

Upledger.com